Kohlhammer

## Die Autorin

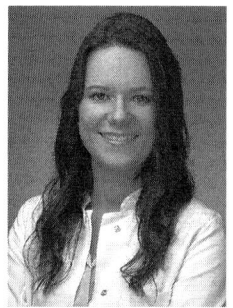

Dr. rer. nat. Jennifer Alexa studierte Pharmazie an der Universität Greifswald. Im Rahmen ihrer Diplomarbeit folgte ein Forschungsaufenthalt an der School of Pharmacy der University of Otago in Neuseeland. Sie ist Fachapothekerin für Arzneimittelinformation, arbeitete in öffentlichen Apotheken in Berlin und promovierte im Bereich der Klinischen Pharmazie an der Universität Leipzig. Während ihrer Auslandsaufenthalte in den U.S.A. und Neuseeland nahm sie an Redeturnieren teil. Zudem leitete sie ein englisches Universitätsdebattierteam in Greifswald und einen Redeclub in Leipzig.

## The author

Dr. Jennifer Alexa studied Pharmacy at the University of Greifswald. While working on her Diploma thesis project, she was a visiting researcher at the University of Otago in New Zealand. She is a specialist pharmacist for drug information, has worked in community pharmacies in Berlin and did her doctoral studies in the field of Clinical Pharmacy at the University of Leipzig. During her stays abroad in the U.S.A. and New Zealand she took part in speech tournaments. She was furthermore the head of the English speaking university debate team in Greifswald and chairwoman of a speech club in Leipzig.

Jennifer Alexa

# Pharmacy Consultation Guide

Englisch für Apotheker und PTAs

2., erweiterte und überarbeitete Auflage

Verlag W. Kohlhammer

Dieses Werk einschließlich aller seiner Teile ist urheberrechtlich geschützt. Jede Verwendung außerhalb der engen Grenzen des Urheberrechts ist ohne Zustimmung des Verlags unzulässig und strafbar. Das gilt insbesondere für Vervielfältigungen, Übersetzungen und für die Einspeicherung und Verarbeitung in elektronischen Systemen.

Pharmakologische Daten verändern sich ständig. Verlag und Autoren tragen dafür Sorge, dass alle gemachten Angaben dem derzeitigen Wissensstand entsprechen. Eine Haftung hierfür kann jedoch nicht übernommen werden. Es empfiehlt sich, die Angaben anhand des Beipackzettels und der entsprechenden Fachinformationen zu überprüfen. Aufgrund der Auswahl häufig angewendeter Arzneimittel besteht kein Anspruch auf Vollständigkeit.

Die Wiedergabe von Warenbezeichnungen, Handelsnamen und sonstigen Kennzeichen berechtigt nicht zu der Annahme, dass diese frei benutzt werden dürfen. Vielmehr kann es sich auch dann um eingetragene Warenzeichen oder sonstige geschützte Kennzeichen handeln, wenn sie nicht eigens als solche gekennzeichnet sind.

Es konnten nicht alle Rechtsinhaber von Abbildungen ermittelt werden. Sollte dem Verlag gegenüber der Nachweis der Rechtsinhaberschaft geführt werden, wird das branchenübliche Honorar nachträglich gezahlt.

Dieses Werk enthält Hinweise/Links zu externen Websites Dritter, auf deren Inhalt der Verlag keinen Einfluss hat und die der Haftung der jeweiligen Seitenanbieter oder -betreiber unterliegen. Zum Zeitpunkt der Verlinkung wurden die externen Websites auf mögliche Rechtsverstöße überprüft und dabei keine Rechtsverletzung festgestellt. Ohne konkrete Hinweise auf eine solche Rechtsverletzung ist eine permanente inhaltliche Kontrolle der verlinkten Seiten nicht zumutbar. Sollten jedoch Rechtsverletzungen bekannt werden, werden die betroffenen externen Links soweit möglich unverzüglich entfernt.

2., erweiterte und überarbeitete Auflage 2024

Alle Rechte vorbehalten
© W. Kohlhammer GmbH, Stuttgart
Gesamtherstellung: W. Kohlhammer GmbH, Stuttgart

Print:
ISBN 978-3-17-041138-8

E-Book-Formate:
pdf: ISBN 978-3-17-041139-5
epub: ISBN 978-3-17-041140-1

# Abkürzungsverzeichnis – List of abbreviations

| | |
|---|---|
| AE | Amerikanisches Englisch |
| BE | Britisches Englisch |
| C | Customer/Kunde |
| etw. | etwas |
| sth. | something |
| GP | General Practitioner |
| ICD/IUCD | intrauterine device/intrauterine contraceptive device |
| i. d. R. | in der Regel |
| inkl. | inklusive/including |
| K | Kunde |
| NPH-Insulin | Neutral Protamin Hagedorn Insulin |
| pl. | Plural/plural |
| POM | prescription-only medicine |
| Rx | Recipere (Latein), bezieht sich in diesem Falle auf verschreibungspflichtige Arzneimittel/Medizinprodukte |
| OTC | over-the-counter |
| S | Sie |
| s. | siehe/see |
| vs. | versus |
| XY | ein beliebiger Begriff/Menge/arbitrary term/quantity |
| Y | You/Sie |

# Inhalt – Content

Abkürzungsverzeichnis – List of abbreviations .................. 5

Übersicht über das elektronische Zusatzmaterial –
Overview of the electronic supplementary material .............. 10

Vorwort – Preface ............................................. 11

Danksagung – Acknowledgements ................................. 14

## I  Basiswissen – Basic Knowledge

**1 Der menschliche Körper – The human body** .................. 17
   1.1   Organsysteme – Organ systems ......................... 17
   1.2   Der Körper – The body ................................ 18
   1.3   Krankheiten/Störungen – Diseases/disorders ........... 19
   1.4   Symptome/Beschwerden – Symptoms/complaints ........... 25

**2 Pharmakologie – Pharmacology** .............................. 30
   2.1   Grundlagen – Basics .................................. 30
   2.2   Wirkstoffklassen – Drug classes ...................... 32

**3 Pharmakotherapie – Pharmacotherapy** ........................ 47
   3.1   Grundbegriffe – General expressions .................. 47
       3.1.1  Produkttyp – Product type ..................... 47
       3.1.2  Arzneimittelinformation – Drug information .... 48
       3.1.3  Pharmakotherapiebezogene Begriffe – Pharmaco-
              therapy-related terms ......................... 48
       3.1.4  Patientengruppe – Patient group ............... 49
   3.2   Darreichungsform – Dosage form ....................... 50
   3.3   Aggregatzustand – Physical form ...................... 52
   3.4   Arzneistoffformulierung – Drug formulation ........... 53
   3.5   Anwendung – Administration ........................... 54
       3.5.1  Applikations-/Anwendungsart – Route of
              administration ................................ 54
       3.5.2  Anwendungshinweise – Administration directions ... 55
       3.5.3  Nebenwirkungen – Side effects ................. 58
       3.5.4  Wechselwirkungen – Interactions ............... 62

|       |       | 3.5.5 Lagerungshinweise – Storage information | 64 |
|---|---|---|---|
|       | 3.6   | Phytotherapie – Phytotherapy | 66 |
|       |       | 3.6.1 Pflanzenteile/Zubereitungen – Plant parts/preparations | 67 |
|       |       | 3.6.2 Tees/Kräuter – Teas/herbals | 68 |
|       | 3.7   | Rezepturen – Pharmaceutical compounding | 71 |
|       | 3.8   | Wundversorgung – Wound treatment | 73 |
|       |       | 3.8.1 Verbandstoffe – Wound dressings | 73 |
|       |       | 3.8.2 Wundarten – Types of wounds | 74 |

## II  Die Beratung – The consultation

**4  Beratungspraxis – Consultation practice** .......... 77
- 4.1 Die Begrüßung – The Greeting .......... 77
- 4.2 Abschlussformeln und Fragen – Finishing phrases and questions .......... 78
- 4.3 Wichtige Fragen und Begriffe – Important questions and terms .......... 78
- 4.4 Selbstmedikation – Self-medication .......... 83
  - 4.4.1 Grenzen der Selbstmedikation – Self-medication limits .......... 85
- 4.5 (Rx) Verschreibungspflichtige Arzneimittel – Prescription only medicines (POMs) .......... 86
  - 4.5.1 Das Rezept – The prescription .......... 87
  - 4.5.2 Rx-Arzneimittel – Prescription only medicines .......... 88

**5  Beratungsthemen – Counseling topics** .......... 92
- 5.1 Erkältung – Common cold .......... 92
  - 5.1.1 Husten – Cough .......... 93
  - 5.1.2 Schnupfen – Stuffy/blocked nose .......... 99
  - 5.1.3 (Kopf-)Schmerzen – Headache/pain .......... 102
- 5.2 Impfungen und Reisekrankheiten – Vaccinations and travel-related diseases .......... 108
- 5.3 Notfallkontrazeption (»Pille danach«) – Emergency contraception (»morning-after pill«/»emergency pill«) .......... 113

**6  Sonstiges – Miscellaneous** .......... 117
- 6.1 Baby-Artikel und -Beschwerden – Baby products and ailments .......... 117
- 6.2 Tierarzneimittel/-artikel – Veterinary medicines/items .......... 118
- 6.3 Fachärzte – Medical specialists .......... 119
- 6.4 Andere Gesundheitsberufe – Other health care professions .......... 120
- 6.5 Die Wochentage – Weekdays .......... 121
- 6.6 Uhrzeiten – Times of the day .......... 122

| III | Nicht pharmazeutische Anliegen – Non-pharmacy related matters | |
|---|---|---|
| 7 | Anliegen und Begriffe – Matters and terms | 125 |
| | 7.1 Wegbeschreibungen – Directions | 125 |
| | 7.2 Nicht pharmazeutische Gegenstände – Non-pharmacy related items | 127 |
| | 7.3 Keine Auskunft möglich – Provision of information not possible | 127 |
| IV | Online-Zusatzmaterial und Wörterverzeichnis – Electronic supplementary material and vocabulary index | |
| 8 | Zusatzmaterial zum Download – Electronic supplementary material | 131 |
| | Wörterverzeichnis – Index | 133 |

# Übersicht über das elektronische Zusatzmaterial – Overview of the electronic supplementary material

Den Weblink, unter dem die Zusatzmaterialien zum Download verfügbar sind, finden Sie unter ▶ Kap. 8 Zusatzmaterial zum Download

You can access the supplementary material via the weblink in chapter 8 Electronic supplementary material

- Übungen 1–4 – Exercises 1–4
- Community Pharmacy Consultation Emergency Card (Übersicht – Overview)

# Vorwort – Preface

Dieses Buch ist eine Orientierungshilfe für das pharmazeutische Beratungsgespräch auf Englisch. Mithilfe von Begriffen, Satzbausteinen und Übungen werden Sie Ihre Kenntnisse vertiefen oder auffrischen können.[1]

Der Inhalt der zweiten erweiterten Auflage dieses Buches gliedert sich in 4 übergeordnete Abschnitte.

Zu Beginn werden Grundlagen der Pharmakologie vorgestellt (▶ Teil I). Anschließend folgen Formulierungshilfen für die pharmazeutische Beratung (▶ Teil II). Abschließend finden Sie Formulierungshilfen für nicht-pharmazeutische Anliegen (▶ Teil III).

Im Online-Zusatzmaterial (▶ Übung 1–4) befinden sich praxisrelevante Übungen und die »Consultation Emergency Card«, welche in kompakter Form einige beratungsrelevante Begriffe, Fragen sowie Floskeln enthält.

Vorab möchte ich Sie darauf hinweisen, dass Englisch je nach Land und Dialekt sehr unterschiedlich sein kann. Aus diesem Grunde wurden an einigen Stellen länderspezifische Redewendungen integriert. Verschiedene Wörter für denselben Begriff können daher auch vorhanden sein. Seien Sie daher nicht verwundert, wenn Ihr U.S.-amerikanischer Kunde[2] nach Acetaminophen statt Paracetamol zur Fiebersenkung fragt. Es kommt nicht darauf an, perfektes Englisch zu sprechen (oftmals ist ihr Gegenüber auch kein »native speaker«), sondern nur Ihrer Beratungspflicht nachgehen zu können. Einige Wirkstoffe und Produkte sind jeweils als Beispiele in kursiver Schrift in Klammern aufgeführt.

**Hinweise zum Tabellenaufbau**

| | |
|---|---|
| **Zwischenüberschriften** | übergeordnete Bezeichnungen in gefetteter Schrift (z. B. übergeordnete Wirkstoffklassen) |
| gleiche farbliche Markierung über mehrere Zeilen | Begriffe/Sätze gehören inhaltlich zusammen |
| *(in kursiver Schrift in Klammern)* | Wirkstoff- oder Produktbeispiele |

---

1 Dieses Buch erhebt keinen Anspruch auf Vollständigkeit. Trotz sorgfältiger Überprüfung können Fehler vorhanden sein. Bei den nachfolgenden Übersetzungen handelt es sich um sinngemäße Übersetzungen, da sich manche Begriffe nicht direkt übersetzen lassen.
2 Aus Gründen der besseren Lesbarkeit wird im Folgenden verallgemeinernd das generische Maskulinum verwendet. Gemeint sind stets alle Geschlechtsformen (weiblich, männlich, divers).

Verbesserungsmöglichkeiten wird es immer geben. Ich freue mich daher über Rückmeldungen zum Buch und/oder Korrekturen via E-Mail (feedback.pharmacy-consultation-guide@skymail.de).
Viel Spaß beim Durchstöbern der nächsten Seiten und viel Erfolg beim nächsten Kundengespräch.

*Jennifer Alexa, im Sommer 2022*

**Preface**

This book serves as a guide for pharmaceutical staff who would like to conduct consultations in English. Content and structure were therefore mainly arranged for German-speaking staff. However, English-speaking staff may also find various German expressions, phrases and excercises helpful for the pharmaceutical consultation.

The content of this second edition is structured into 4 main sections.
In the beginning, fundamentals concerning Pharmacology will be introduced (▶ part I). Subsequently, expressions related to pharmaceutical counseling will be presented (▶ part II). In chapter 3 (▶ part III) you will find expressions concerning non-pharmaceutical matters.
Within the online supplementary material (▶ Exercise 1–4) there are everyday practice-oriented exercises and the »Consultation Emergency Card«, which contains a summary of relevant expressions and phrases.

I would like to point out, that in English as well as in German, the spelling and pronounciation of words may vary locally. Therefore, country-specific expressions in English have been integrated. Do not be confused, if your client from the U.S. for instance inquires about Acetaminophen instead of Paracetamol for fever-reduction. It is not important to speak prefect German (the person in front of you may not be a »native speaker« anyway), but to fullfill your duty to provide information when counseling. Some active ingredients and products are listed as examples in italics in brackets on the following pages.

**Guidance on table structure**

| | |
|---|---|
| subheadings | superordinate terms in bold (e. g. superordinate drug classes) |
| uniform coloring of several lines | terms/sentences belong contentwise together |
| *(in italics in brackets)* | drug or product examples |

There is always room for improvement. I therefore appreciate receiving feedback concerning the book and/or corrections via E-mail (feedback.pharmacy-consultation-guide@skymail.de).
Enjoy reading the following pages and good luck with your next pharmaceutical consultaion.

*Jennifer Alexa, summer of 2022*

# Danksagung – Acknowledgements

Für meine Familie, die mich fortwährend unterstützt hat sowie meine Freunde und Kollegen, insbesondere Irena Albert, die durch konstruktives Feedback zur Konzeption der zweiten Auflage beigetragen haben.

For my family, who continuously supported me as well my friends and colleagues, especially Irena Albert, who provided constructive feedback and therefore helped with conceptualizing the second edition.

Ein besonderer Dank gilt Christopher Gregory und Dr. Geoffrey Smith, die durch ihre Überprüfung einen bedeutenden Beitrag zur Entstehung der zweiten Auflage dieses Buches geleistet haben.

Many thanks goes to Christopher Gregory and Dr. Geoffrey Smith for reviewing this book and therefore making a significant contribution to the creation of the second edition of this book.

# I Basiswissen – Basic Knowledge

# 1 Der menschliche Körper – The human body

## 1.1 Organsysteme – Organ systems

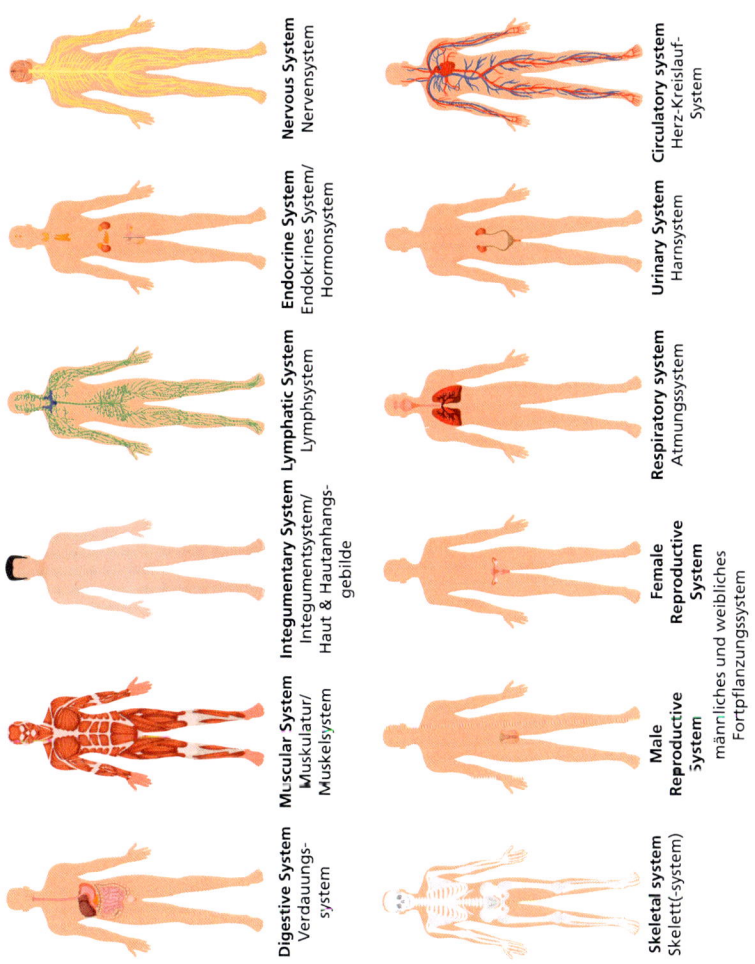

Abb. 1.1: Übersicht der Organsysteme des menschlichen Körpers[3]

---

3 Designed by macrovector/Freepik

I Basiswissen – Basic Knowledge

## 1.2 Der Körper – The body

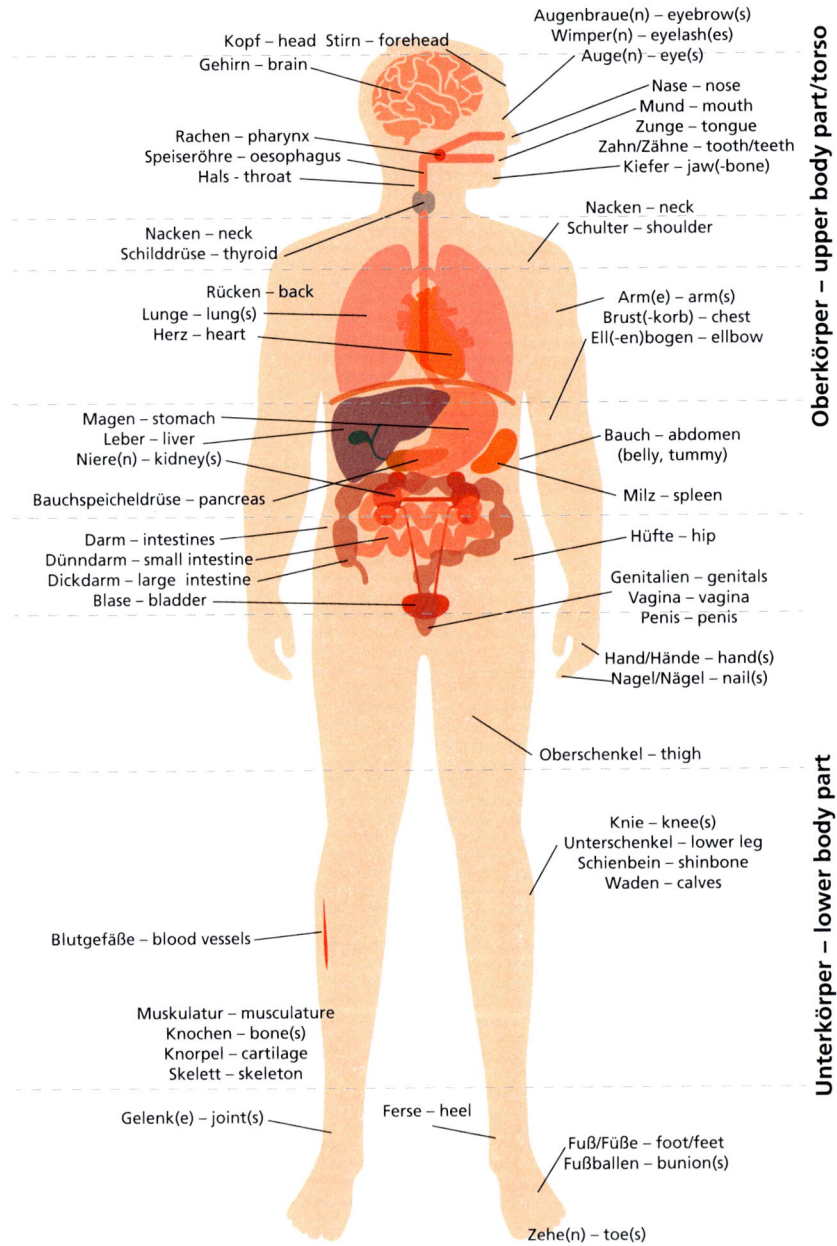

**Abb. 1.2:** Der menschliche Körper[4]

---

4 © iStock | kowalska-art

## 1.3 Krankheiten/Störungen – Diseases/disorders

In den nächsten Tabellen finden Sie eine Auswahl an Krankheiten, Störungen sowie allgemeinen Begriffen, die in diesem Kontext verwendet werden. Überlappungen der Begriffe sind möglich. Einige Krankheiten werden beispielsweise durch mehrere Ursachen ausgelöst (z. B. durch bakterielle Infektionen oder als sekundäre Erkrankung aufgrund einer Primärerkrankung). Sie lassen sich dadurch manchmal in mehrere Bereiche kategorisieren.

Within the tables below you will find a selection of diseases, disorders and general terms that are used in this context. There might be an overlap, since for instance certain diseases may result from various causes (e. g. bacterial infections or as a secondary disease due to a primary disease). They may therefore be classified into several categories.

### Allgemeine Begriffe – General terms

| Krankheit/Erkrankung | disease |
|---|---|
| Leiden/Zustand | condition |
| Störung | disorder |
| bösartig/maligne | malignant/malicious |
| gutartig/benign | benign/good-natured |

### Blutkrankheiten, -störungen und Krankheiten des Immunsystems – Blood/haematological diseases, disorders and diseases of the immune system

| Anämie (z. B. Eisenmangelanämie) | anemia (AE)/anaemia (BE) (e. g. iron deficiency anaemia) |
|---|---|
| Blutgerinnungsstörungen | blood coagulation disorders |
| Leukämie | leukemia (AE)/leukaemia (BE) |
| **Autoimmunerkrankung (Beispiele)** | **autoimmune disease (examples)** |
| Hashimoto-Thyreoiditis | Hashimoto's thyroiditis |
| Lupus erythematodes | lupus erythematosus |
| Psoriasis/Schuppenflechte | psoriasis |
| Zöliakie | celiac disease (AE)/coeliac disease (BE) |

I Basiswissen – Basic Knowledge

## Krankheiten der Atemwege – Diseases of the respiratory tract

| | |
|---|---|
| (akute/chronische) Bronchitis | (acute/chronic) bronchitis |
| Asthma | asthma |
| Atemwegsinfekt | respiratory infection |
| chronisch obstruktive Lungenerkrankung (COPD) | chronic obstructive pulmonary disease (COPD) |
| Rhinitis/Nasenschleimhautentzündung | rhinitis |
| Sinusitis/Nasennebenhöhlenentzündung | sinusitis |

## Erkrankungen im Zusammenhang mit der Ernährung/Begriffe – Nutrition/diet-related diseases/terms

| | |
|---|---|
| Mangel an (z. B. an Vitamin A) | lack of (XY)/deficiency (e. g. vitamin A deficiency) |
| Nahrungsmittel-Allergien | food allergies |
| Übergewicht/Adipositas | obesity/adiposity/adiposis |
| Untergewicht | underweight |

## Hauterkrankungen/-beschwerden – Skin diseases/complaints

| | |
|---|---|
| Akne | acne |
| Dermatitis/Hautentzündung | dermatitis |
| Ekzem | eczema |
| Erythem/Hautrötung | erythema/skin redness |
| Hirsutismus | hirsutism |
| Nesselsucht/Urtikaria | nettle rash/urticaria |
| Neurodermitis | neurodermatitis |
| Rosazea | rosacea |

## Krankheiten/Störungen des Herz-, Kreislaufsystems – Cardiovascular diseases/disorders

| | |
|---|---|
| Angina pectoris/Herzenge | angina pectoris |
| Arrhythmie | arrhythmia |
| Bluthochdruck/Hypertonie | high blood-pressure/hypertension |

1 Der menschliche Körper – The human body

| | |
|---|---|
| niedriger Blutdruck/Hypotonie | low blood pressure/hypotension |
| Embolie | embolism |
| Herzinfarkt/Myokardinfarkt | heart attack/myocardial infarction |
| Herzinsuffizienz | heart failure/cardiac insufficiency |
| Schlaganfall/Hirninfarkt | stroke/seizure |
| Thrombose | thrombosis |
| Vorhofflimmern | atrial fibrilation |

Infektiöse/parasitäre/Pilz-Krankheiten/Befälle – Infectious/parasitic/fungal diseases/infestations

| | |
|---|---|
| Acquired Immune Deficiency Syndrome (AIDS)/Humanes Immundefizienz-Virus (HIV)-Infektion | acquired immune deficiency syndrome (AIDS)/ human immunodeficiency virus (HIV)-infection |
| Borreliose | borreliosis/lyme disease |
| Chikungunya-Fieber | chikungunya virus |
| Cholera | cholera |
| Dengue | dengue |
| Diphtherie | diphtheria |
| Ebolafieber | ebola virus disease (EVD)/ebola hemorrhagic fever (EHF) |
| Flohbefall/Flöhe | flea infestation/fleas |
| Gelbfieber | yellow fever |
| Grippe (die)/Influenza | the flu/influenza |
| hämorrhagisches Fieber | hemorrhagic fever |
| Helicobacter-pylori-Infektion | helicobacter pylori infection |
| Hepatitis | hepatitis |
| Keuchhusten/Pertussis | whooping cough/pertussis |
| Krätze (Skabies) | scabies |
| Lausbefall/Läuse | lice infestation/lice |
| Leishmaniose | leishmaniosis |
| Malaria | malaria |
| Masern | measles |
| Methicillin-resistente Staphylococcus-aureus (MRSA)-Infektion | methicillin-resistant staphylococcus aureus (MRSA)-infection |

I Basiswissen – Basic Knowledge

| Milbenbefall/Milben | mite infestation/mite |
|---|---|
| Mumps | mumps |
| Mundsoor | oral thrush |
| Pest | plague |
| Pilzinfektion/Pilz | fungal infection, mycosis/fungus |
| Scharlach (-fieber) | scarlet fever |
| Sepsis/Blutvergiftung (z. B. durch Streptokokken) | sepsis/blood poisoning (e. g. due to streptococci) |
| Shigellose/Bakterielle Ruhr | shigellosis/bacterial dysentery |
| Syphilis | syphilis |
| Tollwut | rabies |
| Toxoplasmose | toxoplasmosis |
| Tuberkulose | tuberculosis |
| Typhus/Fleckfieber | typhus/typhoid fever |
| Wurmbefall/Helminthosen | worm infestation/helminthiasis |
| Zika | zika |

Krankheiten des Muskel-, Skelett-, Bindehautgewebes – Diseases of the muscular-, skeletal, conjunctival tissue

| Arthritis/Gelenkentzündung | arthritis |
|---|---|
| Arthrose/degenerative Gelenkerkrankung | arthrosis/osteoarthrotis/osteoarthritis/ degenerative joint disease/joint wear |
| Gicht | gout |
| Osteoporose | osteoporosis |

Krankheiten des Nervensystems – Diseases of the nervous system

| Alzheimer-Demenz | Alzheimer's disease/Alzheimer's dementia |
|---|---|
| Enzephalitis/Gehirnentzündung | encephalitis |
| Meningitis/Hirnhautentzündung | meningitis |
| Multiple Sklerose (MS) | multiple sclerosis (MS) |
| Neuropathie(n) | neuropathy/neuropathies |
| Parkinson | Parkinson's disease |

## (Gewebe-) Neubildungen – (tissue) Formation

| | |
|---|---|
| Krebs | cancer |
| Tumor | tumor |

## Erkrankungen/Beschwerden einzelner Organe/Bereiche – Diseases/complaints of certain organs/body parts

| | |
|---|---|
| (Zahn-) Karies | (tooth) caries |
| Aphthe | aphtha/mouth ulcer |
| Blasenentzündung/Zystitis | bladder infection/cystitis |
| Gingivitis/Zahnfleischentzündung | gingivitis/gum inflammation |
| Glaukom/Grüner Star | glaucoma |
| Grauer Star/Katarakt | (eye) cataract |
| Impotenz | impotence |
| Konjunktivitis/Bindehautentzündung | conjunctivitis/eye inflammation |
| Kurzsichtigkeit/Myopie (i. d. R. nicht mit Krankheiten assoziiert, aber der Vollständigkeit halber hier genannt) | short-sightedness/myopia |
| Mandelentzündung | tonsillitis |
| Migräne | migraine |
| Netzhautablösung | retinal detachment |
| Niereninsuffizienz | renal failure/renal insufficiency |
| Parodontitis/Parodontose | parodontitis/periodontitis |
| Prostatahyperplasie | prostate hyperplasia |
| Unfruchtbarkeit | infertility |
| Weitsichtigkeit/Hyperopie (i. d. R. nicht mit Krankheiten assoziiert, aber der Vollständigkeit halber hier genannt) | long-sightedness/hyperopia |

## Psychische Erkrankungen und Verhaltensstörungen – Mental illness and behavioural disorders

| | |
|---|---|
| Depression | depression |
| Panikattacke(n) | panic attack(s) |
| Phobie/eine Phobie haben | phobia/to be phobic |
| Schizophrenie | schizophrenia |

## Stoffwechsel-, endokrine Erkrankungen – Metabolic, endocrine diseases

| | |
|---|---|
| Diabetes (z. B. mellitus) | diabetes (e. g. mellitus) |
| Intoleranz (z. B. Laktoseintoleranz)/ Unverträglichkeit | intolerance (e. g. lactose-intolerance) |
| Mukoviszidose/zystische Fibrose | mucoviscidosis/cystic fibrosis |
| Schilddrüsenüberfunktion/Hyperthyreose | hyperthyroidism |
| Schilddrüsenunterfunktion/Hypothyreose | hypothyroidism |
| Struma | goiter/goitre |

## Krankheiten/Störungen des Verdauungsystems – Diseases/disorders of the digestive system

| | |
|---|---|
| Bauchspeicheldrüsenentzündung/ Pankreatitis | pancreatitis |
| Blinddarmentzündung/(akute) Appendizitis | appendicitis |
| Colitis ulcerosa | ulcerative colitis |
| Gallenblasenentzündung/Cholezystitis | gall baldder inflammation/cholecystitis |
| Gastritis/Magenschleimhautentzündung | gastritis |
| Gastroösophagale Refluxkrankheit (GERD) | gastroesophageal reflux disease (GERD) |
| Leberzirrhose | liver/hepatic cirrhosis |
| Morbus Crohn | Crohn's disease |
| Reizdarmsyndrom | irritable bowel syndrome (IBS) |
| Verdauungsstörung/Dyspepsie | digestive disorder/dyspepsia |

### Beispiel – example

C: I am an insulin-dependent diabetic. Is there anything I need to be aware of before taking the linctus?
Y: Thanks for letting me know. I am happy to check whether it contains sugar.

K: Ich bin ein Insulin-pflichtiger Diabetiker. Gibt es etwas, was ich vor der Einnahme des Hustensaftes beachten sollte?
S: Danke, dass Sie mich darauf hinweisen. Ich schaue gerne für sie nach, ob er Zucker enthält.

## 1.4 Symptome/Beschwerden – Symptoms/complaints

Damit Sie anhand der Schilderung der Symptome Ihres Kunden die richtige Entscheidung treffen können, sind in Kap. 1.4 relevante Begriffe aufgeführt.

In order to make the right decision based on your client's description of their symptoms you will find relevant expressions in chapter 1.4.

### Allgemeine Begriffe – General terms

| | |
|---|---|
| Leiden/Beschwerden (größere/kleinere) | ailment (major/minor) |
| Syndrom | syndrome |
| Symptom | symptom |
| krank (größere Beschwerden) | ill (AE)/major illness (BE)/major ailments |
| krank (leichtere Beschwerden) | sick (AE)/ill; sick (BE)/minor ailments |
| Steigung/Abnahme von XY | increase/decrease in XY |

### Symptombeispiele/Beschwerden – Examples of symptoms/complaints

| | |
|---|---|
| Absonderung | discharge |
| Allergie(n) | allergie(s) |
| allergische Reaktion | allergic reaction |
| Alopezie/Haarausfall | alopecia/hair-loss |
| angeschwollene Lymphknoten | swollen lymph nodes |
| Appetitverlust | loss of appetite |
| Aufstoßen | belching |
| Ausschlag | rash |
| außer Atem sein/geraten | to be out of breath |
| Auswurf (Produktion) | sputum (production) |
| Beckenschmerzen | pelvic pain |
| Benommenheit/benommen sein | light-headedness/to be light-headed |
| Blase/Blasen bekommen | blister/to blister |
| Blindheit/blind sein | blindness/to be blind |
| Blut im Stuhl | blood in stools |

I Basiswissen – Basic Knowledge

| | |
|---|---|
| Blutung | bleeding |
| **Blutdruck** | **blood pressure** |
| Bluthochdruck/Hypertension | high blood pressure/hypertension |
| niedriger Blutdruck/Hypotonie | low blood pressure/hypotension |
| Bradykardie/verlangsamter Herzschlag | bradycardia |
| brüchige Nägel | brittle nails |
| Brustschmerzen | chest pain |
| Cholesterinspiegel (hoher) | (high) cholesterol level |
| Deformierung | deformity |
| Doppeltsehen | double vision |
| Durchfall | diarrhea (AE)/diarrhoea (BE) |
| Durst/durstig sein | thirst/to be thirsty |
| Erbrechen/sich erbrechen/sich übergeben | regurgitation/vomiting/to vomit/to puke |
| Erschöpfung | fatigue |
| Farbveränderung | change in color (AE)/colour (BE) |
| Fehlgeburt | miscarriage |
| Fieber/Fieber haben | fever/to run/have a fever |
| Flatulenz/Blähungen | flatulence |
| Gallensteine | gallstones |
| Geburtswehen | labour pains (AE)/labor pains (BE) |
| gereizte Augen | irritated eyes |
| Geruch/Mundgeruch/schlechter Geruch | odor /odour/(oral)/malodor (AE)/malodour (BE) |
| Gewichtsverlust | loss of weight |
| Gewichtszunahme | weight gain |
| Haarausfall/-verlust | hair loss/loss of hair |
| Halsentzündung | strep throat/inflamed throat |
| Halsweh | sore throat |
| Harnretention/Harnverhalt | urinary retention |
| Hautausschlag/Exanthem | rash/exanthem/exanthema |
| Heiserkeit | hoarseness |
| Herzklopfen/-pochen | (heart/cardiac) palpitation(s) |
| Heuschnupfen | hay fever |

1 Der menschliche Körper – The human body

| | |
|---|---|
| Hörverlust | loss of hearing |
| Hunger/hungrig sein | hunger/to be/feel hungry |
| **Husten** | **cough** |
| trockener (Reiz-)Husten | dry cough |
| produktiver Husten | productive/wet cough |
| Lähmung | paralysis |
| Hyperventilation | hyperventilation |
| Infektion | infection |
| Inkontinenz | incontinence |
| Insektenstich | insect bite/mosquito bite/insect sting |
| Juckreiz/jucken | itch/to itch |
| Kopfschmerzen | headache |
| Krampf/Krämpfe (Schüttelkrampf/-krämpfe; Zuckung/en) | cramp(s) (convulsion(s)) |
| einen Krampf haben | to be seized with a convulsion/cramp/to have a cramp |
| Krampfadern | varicose veins |
| (sich) kratzen | to scratch (oneself) |
| Kribbeln | tingling |
| Lymphknoten (angeschwollene) | (swollen) lymph(atic) gland/nodes |
| Magenblähung | bloating of the stomach |
| Menstruationsbeschwerden/Periodenschmerzen | menstrual complaints/period pain |
| müde/Müdigkeit | tired/tiredness |
| Muskelkrämpfe | muscle cramps |
| Mydriasis/Pupillenerweiterung | mydriasis/pupil dilation |
| Myosis/Pupillenverengung | myosis/pupil constriction |
| Narbe(n) | scar(s) |
| Nasenbluten | epistaxis/nosebleeds |
| Nierensteine | kidney stones |
| niesen | to sneeze |
| Ohnmachtsanfall/Synkope | fainting attack/syncope |
| Ödem/Flüssigkeitsansammlung | edema (AE)/oedema (BE) |
| Ohrenschmerzen | ear-ache/otalgia |

I Basiswissen – Basic Knowledge

| | |
|---|---|
| Pickel | pimple(s) |
| Pilz | fungus |
| Prellung/Bluterguss/Hämatom | bruise/hematoma (AE)/haematoma (BE) |
| hoher/verlangsamter Puls | high/decelerated pulse |
| rauchen/mit dem Rauchen aufhören | to smoke/to quit smoking |
| Reizdarm-Syndrom | irritable bowel syndrome (IBS) |
| (sich) räuspern | to clear one's throat |
| Sättigung | satiety |
| Rückenschmerzen | back pain |
| schläfrig sein/Schlafmangel/Schlaflosigkeit | to be sleepy/lack of sleep/insomnia |
| Schleim/Schleimsekretion/-produktion | mucous (AE)/mucus (BE) secretion |
| Schmerz | pain/ache |
| Schnitt-/Platzwunde/Lazeration | laceration |
| Schuppen | dandruff |
| Schüttelfrost/Zittern | the chills/the shivers/shivering |
| Schwäche/schwach sein/ sich schwach fühlen | weakness/to be/feel weak |
| Schwellung/anschwellen | swelling/to swell |
| Schwindel/schwindelig | dizziness/dizzy |
| Sodbrennen | pyrosis/heartburn |
| Taubheit/taub | numbness/deafness (loss of hearing)/ numb/deaf (loss of hearing) |
| Tachykardie/Herzrasen | tachycardia |
| Tinnitus | tinnitus |
| tränende Augen | watery eyes |
| Tremor/Zucken/Zittern | tremor |
| trockene Haut | dry skin |
| Trockenheit/trocken | dryness/dry |
| Übelkeit/übel sein | nausea/to feel nauseous |
| Verdauungsstörung | dyspepsia |
| verschwitzt sein/Schweiß/in Schweiß ausbrechen | to be sweaty/sweat/perspiration/to break into perspiration |
| verschwommene Sicht | blurred vision |
| verstopfte Nase | stuffy nose/blocked nose |
| Verstopfung | constipation |

| | |
|---|---|
| Völlegefühl/aufgebläht sein | bloating/to feel bloated |
| Warze | verruca/wart |
| Wechseljahrsbeschwerden/menopausale Beschwerden | menopausal complaints/menopausal discomforts |
| Zahnschmerzen | tooth-ache |
| Zeckenbiss | tick bite |

### Beispiel – example

*C: I am not feeling well. I had the chills this morning. Now I also have a sore throat. What would you recommend?*

K: Ich fühle mich nicht gut. Heute Morgen hatte ich Schüttelfrost. Jetzt habe ich zudem Halsweh. Können Sie mir etwas empfehlen?

# 2 Pharmakologie – Pharmacology

## 2.1 Grundlagen – Basics

In Abb. 2.1 sehen Sie einige Begriffe, die im Zusammenhang mit der Pharmakokinetik und -dynamik stehen und auch für die Beratung in der Apotheke relevant sein können.

Figure 2.1 contains some terms that are related to the pharmacokinetics as well as -dynamics and may also be relevant for pharmaceutical counseling.

## 2 Pharmakologie – Pharmacology

### Arzneistoffapplikation – Drug administration

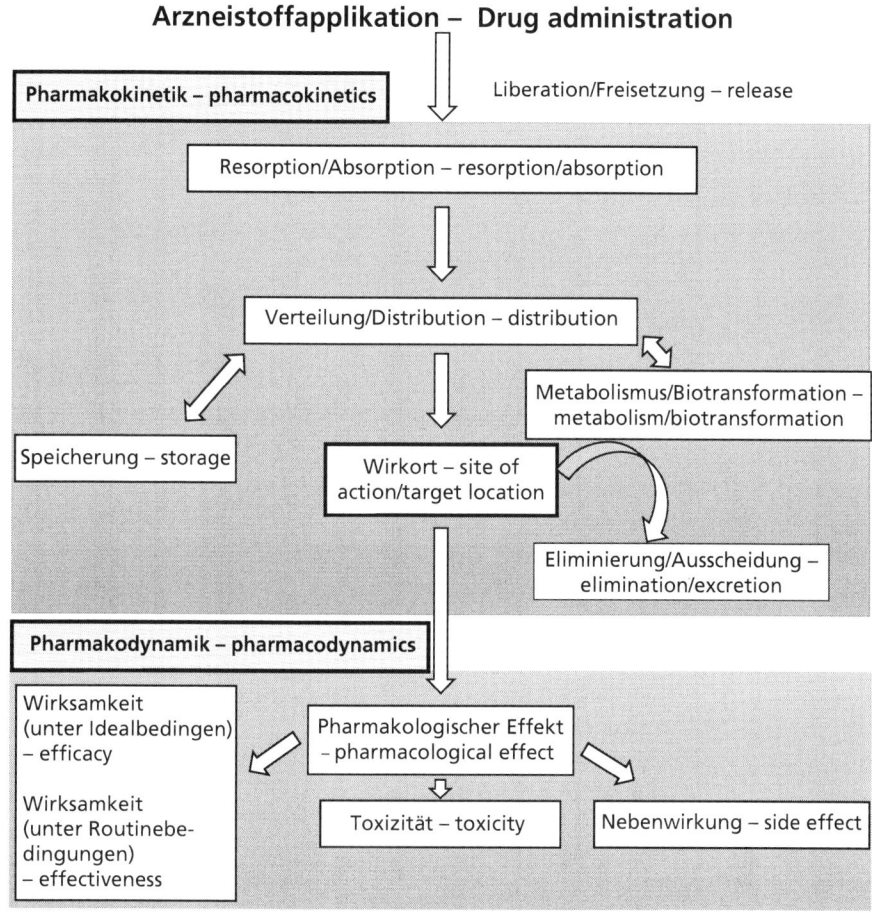

Abb. 2.1: Pharmakologische Grundlagen – Pharmacological basics[5, 6]

### Relevante Begriffe – Relevant terms

| Abbauprodukt | degradation product |
|---|---|
| etw. über die Leber ausscheiden | to excrete sth. via the liver |
| etw. über die Niere ausscheiden | to excrete sth. via the kidneys |
| etw. verstoffwechseln | to metabolize (AE) /to metabolise (BE) sth. |

---

5 Modifiziert nach Pharmacology, Part 2: Introduction to Pharmacokinetics, Currie GM, Journal of Nuclear Medicine TechnologySeptember 2018,46(3)221-230; https://doi.org/10.2967/jnmt.117.199638
6 Fan J, Lannoy de IAM. Pharmacokinetics. Biochem Pharmacol 2014; 87(1): 93–120 https://doi.org/10.1016/j.bcp.2013.09.007

# I Basiswissen – Basic Knowledge

| Gewebe | tissue(s) |
|---|---|
| Körperflüssigkeiten | body fluid(s) |
| Löslichkeit/löslich | solubility/soluble |
| lipophil | lipophilic/lipophil |
| hydrophil | hydrophilic/hydrophil |
| Metabolit(e) | metabolite(s) |

**Beispiel – example**

*Ibuprofen is an analgesic, which is mainly excreted via the kidneys.*
Ibuprofen ist ein Analgetikum, welches hauptsächlich über die Niere ausgeschieden wird.

## 2.2 Wirkstoffklassen – Drug classes

In Kap. 2.2 werden Wirkstoffklassen mit den jeweiligen Vertretern in alphabetischer Reihenfolge aufgeführt. In beiden Spalten finden Sie auch jeweils einen Wikrstoffvertreter in kursiver Schrift in den Klammern. Übergeordnete Wirkstoffklassen sind in fett markiert. Für manche Substanzklassen exisitieren mehrere Namen und sie lassen sich manchmal mehreren Wirkstoffklassen zuordnen. Einige der aufgeführten Substanzen unterliegen der Verschreibungspflicht.

In chapter 2.2 drug classes and associated substances are listed in alphabetical order. Example active ingredients are listed in italics in both columns in brackets. The main drug classes are printed in bold letters. There are several names for some of the substance classes and some may be assigned to several drug classes. Some of these substances are prescription-only substances.

### Analgetika/Schmerzmittel – Analgesics/painkiller

| | |
|---|---|
| **Nicht-Opioid-Analgetika** *(Paracetamol)* | **non-opoid analgesics** *(Acetaminophen (AE)/Paracetamol)* |
| nicht-steroidale Antiphlogistika (NSAIDs) *(Ibuprofen)* | non-steroidal anti-inflammatory drugs/antiphlogistics (NSAIDs) *(Ibuprofen)* |
| **Opioid-Analgetika** *(Morphin)* | **opioid analgesics** *(Morphine)* |

## 2 Pharmakologie – Pharmacology

### Antazida – Antacids/agents reducing acidity

| | |
|---|---|
| **Histamin-2-Antagonisten**/H₂-Antihistaminika (*Ranitidin*) | **histamine-2 antagonists**/H₂-antihistamines (*Ranitidine*) |
| **ionenhaltige Verbindungen** (*Natriumhydrogencarbonat*) | **ionic compounds** (*Sodium hydrogen carbonate*) |
| **Protonenpumpeninhibitoren** (PPIs) (*Pantoprazol*) | **proton pump inhibitors** (*Pantoprazole*) |

### Anthelminthika/»Wurmmittel« (*Pyrvinium*) – Antihelminthics/vermicide/vermifugal (*Pyrvinium*)

### Antiallergika – Antiallergics

| | |
|---|---|
| **Antihistaminika** (*Loratadin*) | **antihistamines** (*Loratadine*) |
| **Antikörper** (z. B. Anti-IgE-Antikörper) (*Omalizumab*) | **antibodies** (e. g. anti-IgE antibodies) (*Omalizumab*) |
| **Hyposensibilisierung**/spezifische Immuntherapie (SIT) (*Lais®*) | **hyposensitization** (AE)/hyposensitisation (BE)/specific immunotherapy (SIT) (*Lais®*) |
| **Leukotrien-Antagonisten** (*Montelukast*) | **anti-leukotrienes** (*Montelukast*) |
| **Mastzellstabilisatoren** (*Cromoglicinsäure*) | **mast cell stabilizers** (*Cromoglicic acid*) |
| (Beta-2-/ß-2-)**Sympathomimetika** (*Salbutamol*) | (beta-2-/ß-2-)**sympathomimetics** (*Salbutamol*) |

### Antidementiva/Nootropika – Antidementives/antidementia drugs/agents/nootropics

| | |
|---|---|
| **Acetylcholinesterasehemmer** (*Rivastigmin*) | **acetylcholinesterase inhibitors** (*Rivastigmine*) |
| **N-Methyl-D-Aspartat** (NMDA)-**Rezeptorantagonisten** (*Memantin*) | **N-methyl-D-aspartate** (NMDA)-**receptor antagonists** (*Memantine*) |
| **Phytotherapeutika** (*Ginkgo-biloba-Extrakt*) | **phytotherapeutics** (*Gingko biloba extract*) |

### Antidepressiva – Antidepressants

| | |
|---|---|
| **Monoaminooxidase**-(MAO-) **Inhibitoren**/Hemmer (*Moclobemid*) | **monoamine oxidase** (MAO-) **inhibitors**/blockers (*Moclobemide*) |
| **selektive Noradrenalin-Dopamin-Reuptake/Wiederaufnahme-Hemmer** (*Bupropion*) | **selective noradrenaline dopamine reuptake inhibitors** (*Bupropion*) |

I Basiswissen – Basic Knowledge

| | |
|---|---|
| selektive Noradrenalin-Reuptake/Wiederaufnahme-Hemmer (Reboxetin) | selective noradrenaline reuptake inhibitors (Reboxetine) |
| selektive Serotonin-/Noradrenalin-Reuptake-/Wiederaufnahme-Hemmer (Venlafaxin) | selective serotonin noradrenaline reuptake inhibitors (Venlafaxine) |
| selektive Serotonin-Reuptake/Wiederaufnahme-Hemmer (SSRI) (Fluoxetin) | selective serotonin reuptake inhibitors (SSRI) (Fluoxetine) |
| tetrazyklische Antidepressiva (Maprotilin) | tetracyclic antidepressants (Maprotiline) |
| $α_2$-Antagonisten (Mirtazapin) | $α_2$-adrenoceptor antagonists (Mirtazapine) |
| trizyklische Antidepressiva (Amitriptylin) | tricyclic antidepressants (Amitriptyline) |
| **sonstige (Auswahl)** | **others (selection)** |
| Melatonin-Rezeptor-Agonisten (Agomelatin) | melatonin agonists (Agomelatine) |
| Phytotherapeutika (Johanniskraut-Extrakt) | phytotherapeutics (St. John's Wort extract) |

Antidiabetika/blutglukosesenkende Arzneimittel – Antidiabetics/blood glucose lowering drug(s)

| Insulin(e) | insulin(s) |
|---|---|
| rasch wirksame Insuline (Insulin lispro – Humalog®) | rapid-acting insulins (Insulin lispro – Humalog®) |
| kurz wirksame Insuline (Humaninsulin – Actrapid®) | short-acting insulins (Human insulin – Actrapid®) |
| intermediär wirksame Insuline/Verzögerungsinsulin (Insulin-Isophan (NPH) – Protaphane®) | intermediate-acting insulins (human isophane (NPH) Insulin – Protaphane®) |
| lang wirksame Insuline (Insulin glargin – Lantus®) | long-acting insulins (glargine Insulin – Lantus®) |
| Mischinsulin (Actraphane®) | mixed insulins (Actraphane®) |
| **Zubehör** | **equipment** |
| Insulinpen | insulin pen |
| Insulinpumpe | insulin pump |
| Insulinspritze | insulin syringe |
| **orale Antidiabetika** | **oral antidiabetics** |
| α-Glukosidasehemmer (Acarbose) | α-glucosidase inhibitors (Acarbose) |
| **Biguanide** (Metformin) | **biguanides** (Metformin) |
| Gliflozine/Natrium-abhängige Glukose-Kotransporter-2 (SGLT-2-)-Inhibitoren (Canagliflozin) | glifozins/sodium dependent glucose co-transporter 2-(SGLT-2-) inhibitors (Canagliflozin) |

| orale Antidiabetika | oral antidiabetics |
|---|---|
| Glinide/Sulfonylharnstoffanaloga (Repaglinid) | glinides/sulfonylurea-analogues (Repaglinide) |
| Glitazone/Insulin-Sensitizer/Peroxisom-Proliferator-aktivierte Rezeptoren γ (PPARγ)-Agonisten (Rosiglitazon) | glitazones/insulin sensitizer/peroxisome proliferator-activated receptor γ (PPARγ-) agonists (Rosiglitazone) |
| Inkretinmimetika (Liraglutid) | incretin mimetics (Liraglutide) |
| Sulfonylharnstoffe (Glibenclamid) | sulfonylureas (Glibenclamide) |
| Gliptine/Dieptidyl-Peptidase-4 (DPP-4)-Inhibitoren (Sitagliptin) | gliptins/Inhibitors of dipeptidyl peptidase 4 (DPP-4) inhibitors (Sitagliptin) |

Antidiarrhoika – Antidiarrheals (AE)/antidiarrhoeals (BE)

| Antipropulsiva/Peristaltikhemmer (Loperamid) | antipropulsives (Loperamide) |
|---|---|
| Elektrolyte/orale salzhaltige Rehydrationsformulierungen (Elotrans®-Pulver) | electrolytes/oral rehydration salt formulations (Elotrans®-powder) |
| mikrobielle Antidiarrhoika: s. Probiotika – microbiological antidiarrhoics: s. probiotics | |
| Antibiotika (Rifaximin) | antibiotics (Rifaximin) |
| Enkephalinase-Inhibitoren (Racecadotril) | enkephalinase inhibitors (Racecadotril) |
| Adsorbenzien (Aktiv-Kohle) | adsorbents (Activated coal) |
| Adstringenzien (Tannin-Albuminat) | astringents (Tannin albuminate) |
| Quellstoffe (Flohsamenschalen) | swelling agents (Psyllium husk) |
| (eingestellte) Opiumtinktur | opium tincture |

Antidote/Antitoxine (Physostigmin) – Antidots/antitoxins (Physostigmine)

Antiemetika – Antiemetics

| s. Antihistaminika – antihistamines | |
|---|---|
| Ingwer(-wurzelstock) | (rootstock of) ginger |
| Serotonin 5-HT₃-Rezeptor-Antagonisten (Ondansetron) | serotonin 5-HT₃ antagonists (Ondansetron) |
| Prokinetika (Metoclopramid) | prokinetics (Metoclopramide) |
| Neuoleptika (Droperidol) | neuroleptics (Droperidol) |
| Neurokinin-Rezeptor-1-Antagonisten (Aprepitant) | neurokinin-1 receptor antagonists (Aprepitant) |

## Antiinfektiva – Antiinfectives

| Antibiotikum/Antibiotika | antibiotic(s) |
| --- | --- |
| Aminoglykoside (*Gentamicin*) | aminoglycoside(s) (*Gentamicin*) |
| **ß-Lactam-Antibiotika** | **ß-lactam antibiotic(s)** |
| Carbapeneme (*Meropenem*) | carbapenems (*Meropenem*) |
| Cephalosporine (*Cefuroxim*) | cephalosporins (*Cefuroxime*) |
| Monobactame (*Aztreonam*) | monobactams (*Aztreonam*) |
| Penicilline (*Amoxicillin*) | penicillins (*Amoxicillin*) |
| ß-Laktamase-Inhibitoren (*Clavulansäure*), der Vollständigkeit halber an dieser Stelle erwähnt, keine Wirkstoffklasse, sondern nur ein Zusatz zur Verhinderung der Antibiotikainaktivierung | ß-lactamase inhibitors (*Clavulanic acid*), only mentioned here for the sake of completeness, this is no drug class of its own, but used as an additive to prevent antibiotic inactivation |
| *Chloramphenicol* | *Chloramphenicol* |
| **Glykopeptide** (*Vancomycin*) | **glycopeptides** (*Vancomycin*) |
| Gyrasehemmer/Fluorchinolone (*Ciprofloxacin*) | gyrase inhibitor(s)/fluoroquinolones (*Ciprofloxacin*) |
| Lincosamide (*Clindamycin*) | lincosamides (*Clindamycin*) |
| Makrolide (*Azithromycin*) | macrolides (*Azithromycin*) |
| *Metronidazol* | *metronidazole* |
| Polypeptidantibiotika (*Bacitracin*) | polypeptide antibiotics (*Bacitracin*) |
| Oxizolidinone (*Linezolid*) | oxizolidinones (*Linezolid*) |
| Sulfonamide/Diaminopyrimidine (*Sulfamethoxazol*) | sulphonamides/diaminopyrimidine antibiotics (*Sulfamethoxazole*) |
| Tetrazykline (*Doxyzyklin*) | tetracyclins (*Doxycycline*) |
| sonstige (*Fosfomycin*) | others (*Fosfomycin*) |
| **Glukokortikoide** – glucocorticosteroids: s. Steroidhormone – steroid hormones | |

## Antimigräne-Mittel – Antimigraine agents

| | |
| --- | --- |
| s. **Analgetika** – analgetics | |
| s. **Antiemetika** – antiemetics | |
| Triptane/Serotonin 5-HT$_{1B/1D}$-Agonisten (*Sumatriptan*) | triptans/serotonin 5-HT$_{1B/1D}$-agonists (*Sumatriptan*) |
| **In der Prophylaxe** | **for prophylaxis** |
| Antiepileptika (*Topiramat*) | antiepileptics (*Topiramate*) |

| | |
|---|---|
| Beta-Blocker (*Metoprolol*) | beta-blockers (*Metoprolol*) |
| Kalziumantagonisten (*Flunarizin*) | calcium antagonists (*Flunarizine*) |
| Calcitonin-Gene-Related-Peptide (CGRP)-Inhibitoren (monoklonale Antikörper, *Erenumab*) | Calcitonin-Gene-Related-Peptide (CGRP)-inhibitors (monoclonal antibodies, *Erenumab*) |
| Muskelrelaxanzien (BOTOX®) | muscle relaxants (BOTOX®) |
| trizyklische Antidepressiva (*Amitryptilin*) | tricyclic antidepressants (*Amitryptiline*) |

## Antimykotika – Antimycotics/antifungals

| | |
|---|---|
| **Allylamin(e)**/Squalenepoxidasehmmer (*Terbinafin*) | **allylamine antifungals**/squalene epoxidase inhibitors (*Terbinafine*) |
| **Azol-Antimykotika** (*Fluconazol*) | **azole antifungals** (*Fluconazole*) |
| **Echocandine** (*Caspofungin*) | **echocandins** (*Caspofungin*) |
| **Mitosehemmer** (*Griseofulvin*) | **mitosis inhibitors** (*Griseofulvin*) |
| **Morpholin-Derivat(e)** (*Amorolfin*) | **morpholine antifungals** (*Amorolfine*) |
| **Polyen(e)** (*Nystatin*) | **polyene antifungals** (*Nystatin*) |
| sonstige (*Ciclopirox*) | others (*Ciclopirox*) |

## Anti-inflammatorische Mittel/Antiphlogistika/Entzündungshemmer – Anti-inflammatory agents

| | |
|---|---|
| Antikörper (*Adalimumab*) | antibodies (*Adalimumab*) |
| s. NSAIDs und Glukokortikosteroide – s. NSAIDs and glucocorticosteroids | |

## Antithrombose-Mittel – Antithrombotic agents

| | |
|---|---|
| Antifibrinolytika (*Tranexamsäure*) | antifibrinolytics (*Tranexamic acid*) |
| **Antikoagulantien** | **anticoagulants** |
| direkte Thrombininhibitoren (*Dabigatran*) | direct thrombin inhibitors (*Dabigatran*) |
| direkte Faktor-Xa-Hemmer (*Apixaban*)/ auch direkte orale Antikoagluatien (DOAK), neue orale Antikoagulantien (NOAK) genannt | direct factor Xa (FXa) inhibitors (*Apixaban*) |
| indirekte Faktor-Xa-Hemmer (*Fondaparinux*) | indirect factor Xa inhibitors (*Fondaparinux*) |
| Heparin(e) (*Enoxaparin*) | heparin(s) (*Enoxaparin*) |

| | |
|---|---|
| Vitamin-K-Antagonist(en) (*Phenprocoumon*) | vitamin-K-antagonist(s) (*Phenprocoumon*) |
| Fibrinolytika (*Alteplase*) | fibrinolytics (*Alteplase*) |
| **Thrombozytenfunktionshemmer/Thrombozytenaggregationshemmer** | **platelet inhibitors/platelet aggregation inhibitors** |
| Adenosindiphosphat (ADP)-Rezeptor-Antagonisten (*Clopidogrel*) | adenosine diphosphate (ADP)-receptor antagonists (*Clopidogrel*) |
| Cyclooxygenasehemmer (*Acetylsalicylsäure*) | Cyclooxygenase inhibitors (*Acetylsalicylic acid*) |
| Glykoprotein (GP)-IIb/IIIa-Antagonisten (*Eptifibatid*) | Glycoprotein (GP) IIb-IIIa antagonists (*Eptifibatide*) |
| Phosphodiesterase-III (PDE-3)-Hemmer (*Cilostazol*) | Phosphodiesterase-III (PDE3)-inhibitors (*Cilostazol*) |

## Antihämorrhagische Mittel/Antihämorrhagika/blutstillende Mittel – Antihaemorrhagic agents

| | |
|---|---|
| Blutgerinnungsfaktoren (*Faktor VIII*) | blood coagulation factors/blood clotting factors (*factor VIII*) |
| Vitamin K | Vitamin K |

## Antianämika – Antianemic preparations

| | |
|---|---|
| eisenhaltige Produkte (*Ferro Sanol®*) | iron products (*Ferro Sanol®*) |

## Anästhetika – Anesthetics (AE)/anaesthetics (BE)

| | |
|---|---|
| Lokalanästhetika (*Lidocain*) | local anaesthetics (*Lidocaine*) |
| **Inhalationsanästhetika** (*Sevofluran*) | **inhalational/volatile anaesthetics** (*Sevoflurane*) |
| **Injektionsanästhetika** (*Propofol*) | **injectable anaesthetics** (*Propofol*) |

## Antiepileptika/Antikonvulsiva – Anticonvulsive agents/antiepileptics

Die Klassifikation der Antikonvulsiva basiert i. d. R. auf der pharmakologischen Wirkung anstelle der chemischen Struktur.

The classification of anticonvulsives is usually based on their pharmacological effect instead of the chemical structure.

| | |
|---|---|
| Carboanhydrasehemmer (*Sultiam*) | carbonic anhydrase inhibitors (*Sultiame*) |
| **Blockade spannungsabhängiger Kalzium-/ Natriumkanäle** (*Valproat*) | **blockage of voltage-dependent calcium/sodium channels** (*Valproate*) |
| Wirkverstärkung des inhibitorischen Neurotransmitters γ-Aminobuttersäure (GABA) (*Levetiracetam*) | effect amplification of the inhibitory neurotransmitter γ-aminobutyric acid (GABA) (*Levetiracetam*) |
| **sonstige** z. B. Wirkhemmung exzitatorischer (»stimulierender«) Neurotransmitter wie Glutamat (*Topiramat*) | **others** e. g. effect inhibition of excitatory (»stimulating«) neurotransmitters such as glutamate (*Topiramate*) |

## Antiparkinsonmittel – Antiparkinson drugs

| | |
|---|---|
| Dopamin-$D_2$-Rezeptoragonisten (*Pramipexol*) | dopamine $D_2$-receptor agonists (*Pramipexole*) |
| *Levodopa/L-Dopa* wird in der Regel mit Decarboxylase-Hemmern (*Carbidopa*) oder Catechol-O-Methyl-Transferase (COMT)-Hemmern (*Entacapon*) gegeben, um den Abbau von L-Dopa in der Peripherie zu blockieren | *Levodopa/L-Dopa* is usually given in combination with decarboxylase inhibitors (*Carbidopa*) or catechol-O-methyl-transferase (COMT)-inhibitors (*Entacapon*) in order to prevent the peripheral breakdown of L-Dopa |
| **Monoaminooxidase (MAO)-B-Hemmer** (*Rasagilin*) | **monoamine oxidase (MAO) B-inhibitors** (*Rasagiline*) |
| **Muskarinrezeptorantagonisten** (MRA, *Biperiden*) | **muscarinic receptor antagonists** (MRA, *Biperiden*) |
| **N-Methyl-D-Aspartat (NMDA)-Rezeptorantagonisten** (*Amantadin*) | **N-methyl-D-aspartate (NMDA)-receptor antagonists** (*Amantadine*) |

Antipyretika/fiebersenkendes Mittel (*Ibuprofen*) – Antipyretics (*Ibuprofen*)

Antiseptika (*Povidon-Iod*) – Antiseptics (*Povidon-Iod*)

Anxiolytika – Anxiolytics

| | |
|---|---|
| Antipsychotika/Neuroleptika (*Pregabalin*) | antipsychotics/neuroleptics (*Pregabalin*) |
| **Barbiturate** (*Phenobarbital*, obsolet!) | **barbiturates** (*Phenobarbital*, obsolete!) |
| Benzodiazepine (*Diazepam*) | benzodiazepines (*Diazepam*) |
| Phytotherapeutika (*Lavendelöl*) | phytotherapeutics (*Lavender oil*) |
| s. Antidepressiva/Beta-Blocker/Antiepileptika | s. antidepressants/beta-blockers/antiepileptics |

I Basiswissen – Basic Knowledge

## Digestiva/verdauungsfördernde Mittel – Digestives

| Cholagoga/»Gallemittel« | cholagogues/«bile remedies« |
|---|---|
| Cholekinetika (Sorbitol) | cholekinetics (Sorbitol) |
| Choleretika (Artischockenblätter) | choleretics (Artichoke leaves) |
| **Bittermittel/Amara** (Enzian) | **(digestive) bitters** (gentian) |
| **Prokinetika** (Domperidon) | **prokinetics** (Domperidone) |
| **Enzym-Präparate (Lipase)** | **Enzymes (Lipase)** |

## Gichttherapie-Arzneimittel – Gout therapy agents

| *Colchicin* | *Colchicine* |
|---|---|
| **Urikolytika** (Rasburicase) | **uricolytics** (Rasburicase) |
| **Urikostatika** (Allopurinol) | **uricostatics** (Allopurinol) |
| **Urikosurika** (Probenecid) | **uricosurics** (Probenecid) |
| **nicht-steroidale Antiphlogistika/Antirheumatika** (NSAIDs) (Diclofenac) | **non-steroidal anti-inflammatory drugs/antiphlogistics** (NSAIDs) (Diclofenac) |

## Hepatika/Lebertherapeutika – Liver therapeutics

| (L-)Ornithin(L-)aspartat | (L-)Ornithine(L-)Aspartate |
|---|---|
| **lipotrope Substanzen** (Mariendistelfrüchte) | **lipotropics** (milk thistle fruits) |

## Immunsuppressiva – Immunosuppressants/immunosuppressives

| Antikörper (z. B. Tumornekrosefaktor-alpha (TNF-α)-Inhibitoren) (Adalimumab) | antibodies (e. g. tumor necrosis factor alpha (TNF-α)-inhibitors) (Adalimumab) |
|---|---|
| **s. Glukokortikoide – glucocorticoids** | |
| **Calcineurininhibitoren** (Ciclosporin) | **calcineurin inhibitors** (Cyclosporine) |
| **selektive Serin-/Threonin-Kinase-Inhibitoren** (mTOR-Inhibitoren) (Sirolimus) | **serine/threonine-specific protein kinase inhibitors** (mechanistic target of rapamycin, mTOR) (Sirolimus) |
| **Kostimulationsblocker** (Belatacept) | **Co-stimulation blocker** (Belatacept) |
| **Antimetabolite** (Azathioprin) | **antimetabolites** (Azathioprine) |
| einige Zytostatika, some cytostatics: s. **Zytostatika – cytostatics** | |

## Herz-Kreislauf-Mittel – Cardiovascular agents

| Antiarrhythmika | antiarrhythmics |
|---|---|
| Betablocker (Bisoprolol) | beta-blocking agents/beta-blockers (Bisoprolol) |
| Digitalisglykoside (Digoxin) | digitalis glycosides (Digoxin) |
| Kaliumkanalblocker (Amiodaron) | potassium channel blockers (Amiodarone) |
| Kalziumantagonisten/Kalziumkanalblocker (Diltiazem) | calcium channel antagonists/calcium channel blockers (Diltiazem) |
| Natriumkanalblocker (Flecainid) | sodium channel blockers (Flecainide) |
| **Antihypertensiva/Antihypertonika** | **antihypertensives/blood pressure lowering agents** |
| Angiotensin-Konversionsenzym (ACE)-Hemmer/ACE-Inhibitoren (Ramipril) | angiotensin-converting enzyme (ACE)-inhibitors/ACE-inhibitors (Ramipril) |
| Sartane/AT$_1$-Rezeptorantagonisten (Valsartan) | sartan family/AT$_1$-receptor antagonists (Valsartan) |
| s. Betablocker/beta-blocking agents | |
| **Diuretika** | **diuretics** |
| Carboanhydrase-Inhibitoren (Acetazolamid) | carbonic anhydrase inhibitors (Acetazolamide) |
| Thiazid-Diuretika (Hydrochlorothiazid) | thiazide-diuretics (Hydrochlorothiazide) |
| Schleifendiuretika (Furosemid) | loop diuretics (Furosemide) |
| kaliumsparende Diuretika (Triamteren) | potassium-sparing diuretics (Triamteren) |
| Aldosteron-Antagonisten (Eplerenon) | aldosterone antagonists (Eplerenone) |
| Vasopressin-Rezeptor-Antagonisten/Vaptane (Tolvaptan): Zur Behandlung von Hyponatriämien eingesetzt, der Vollständigkeit halber hier erwähnt | vasopressin receptor antagonists/vaptans (Tolvaptan): used to treat hyponatremia, only mentioned here for the sake of completeness |
| osmotische Diuretika (Glycerin) | osmotic diuretics (Glycerine) |
| s. Kalziumantagonisten/Kalziumkanalblocker (Amlodipin) – calcium channel antagonists/calcium channel blockers (Amlodipine) | |
| Renin-Inhibitoren (Aliskiren) | renin inhibitors (Aliskiren) |
| **Vasodilatatoren** | **vasodilatators** |
| Nitrate/Stickstoffmonoxid (NO)-Donatoren (Nitroglycerin) | nitrates/nitrogen monoxide (NO)-donators (Nitroglycerin) |
| andere (Minoxidil) | others (Minoxidil) |

## Hormone – Hormones

| | |
|---|---|
| **Gewebshormone** (*Serotonin/5-Hydroxytryptamin/5-HT*)<br>In der Therapie werden z. B. Serotonin-5-HT-Agonisten und -Antagonisten eingesetzt (*Metoclopramid*). | **tissue hormones** (*Serotonin/5-Hydroxytryptamine/5-HT*)<br>serotonine 5-HT-agonists and -antagonists are being used for therapy/treatment (*Metoclopramide*). |
| **Hormone der Nebennierenrinde** | **hormones of the adrenal cortex** |
| Glukokortikoide (*Prednison*) | glucocorticoids (*Prednisone*) |
| Mineralkortikoide (*Aldosteron*) | mineralocorticoids (*Aldosterone*) |
| **Sexualhormone** | **reproductive hormones/sex hormones** |
| Androgene (*Testosteron*) | androgens (*Testosterone*) |
| Antiandrogene (*Apalutamid*) | antiandrogens (*Apalutamide*) |
| Antiestrogene (*Tamoxifen*) | antiestrogens (*Tamoxifen*) |
| Estrogene/Östrogene (*Ethinylestradiol*) | estrogens (*Ethinylestradiol*) |
| Gestagene (*Levonorgestrel*) | gestagens (*Levonorgestrel*) |
| Gonadotropin-Releasing Hormone (GnRH)-Analoga (*Buserelin*) | gonadotropin releasing hormone (GnRH)-analogues (*Buserelin*) |
| Gonadotropin-Releasing Hormone (GnRH)-Antagonisten (*Degarelix*) | gonadotropin-releasing hormone (GnRH)-antagonists (*Degarelix*) |

## Karminativa (*Kümmel*) – Carminatives (*caraway*)

## Laxanzien – Laxatives

| | |
|---|---|
| osmotisch wirksame Laxanzien (*Lactulose*) | osmotically active laxatives (*Lactulose*) |
| **Quellmittel** (*Leinsamen*) | **swelling agents** (*linseed*) |
| **Klysmen/Einläufe** (*Glycerol*) | **enemas** (*glycerin (AE)/glycerine (BE)*) |
| **salinische Laxanzien** (*Magnesiumsulfat/Bittersalz*) | **salin laxatives** (*magnesium sulfate/Epsom salt*) |
| **Antiresorptive/sekretagoge Laxanzien** | **antiresorptive/secretagogue laxatives** |
| Diphenole (*Natriumpicosulfat*) | diphenols (*Sodium picosulfate*) |
| *Rizinusöl* | *Castor oil* |
| Anthrachinon-Derivate (*Rhabarber*) | anthraquinone derivatives (*Rhubarb*) |
| **andere** | **others** |
| Prokinetika/Serotonin (5-HT$_4$)-Rezeptoragonisten (*Prucaloprid*) | prokinetics/serotonin (5-HT$_4$)-receptor agonists (*Prucalopride*) |

| Guanylatcyclase-C-Rezeptoragonisten (*Linaclotid*) | guanylate cyclase-C agonists (*Linaclotide*) |
| --- | --- |
| peripher wirksame Opioid-Rezeporantagonisten (*Methylnaltrexon*) | peripherally acting opoid receptor antagonists (*Methylnaltrexone*) |

## Lipidsenker/Antilipidämika – Lipid-lowering drug/lipid reducers/antihyperlipidemics

| | |
| --- | --- |
| **Fibrate** (*Fenofibrat*) | **fibrates** (*Fenofibrate*) |
| **Statine/HMG-CoA-Reduktase-Inhibitoren** (*Simvastatin*) | **statins**/HMG-CoA reductase inhibitors (*Simvastatin*) |
| **Cholesterol-Resorptionshemmer** (*Ezetimib*) | **cholesterol absorption inhibitors** (*Ezetimibe*) |
| **Ionenaustauscherharze** (*Colesytramin*) | **ion exchange resins** (*Colesytramine*) |
| Nikotinsäure (*obsolet!*) | nicotinic acid (*obsolete!*) |
| **Phytotherapeutika** (*Artischocke*) | **phytotherapeutics** (*artichoke*) |
| **Antikörper** (*Alirocumab*) | **antibodies** (*Alirocumab*) |

## Mineralstoffe – Minerals/mineral substances

| | |
| --- | --- |
| *Eisen* | *iron* |
| *Fluorid* | *fluoride* |
| *Jod* | *iodine* |
| *Kalium* | *potassium* |
| *Kalzium* | *calcium* |
| *Kieselerde* | *silica* |
| *Kupfer* | *copper* |
| *Magnesium* | *magnesium* |
| *Natrium* | *sodium* |
| *Selen* | *selenium* |
| *Silicium* | *silicon* |
| *Zink* | *zinc* |

I Basiswissen – Basic Knowledge

## Osteoporose-Mittel – Osteoporosis treatment agents

| | |
|---|---|
| **Bisphosphonate** (*Alendronsäure*) | **bisphosphonates** (*Alendronic acid*) |
| **Parathormon-Analoga** (*Teriparatid*) | **parathyroid hormone analogues** (*Teriparatide*) |
| **Antikörper**/receptor activator of nuclear factor kappa-B (NF-κB) ligand (RANKL)-Inhibitoren (*Denosumab*) | **antibodies**/receptor activator of nuclear factor kappa-B (NF-κB) ligand (RANKL)-inhibitors (*Denosumab*) |
| **selektive Estrogenrezeptor-Modulatoren (SERMs)** (*Raloxifen*) | **selective estrogen receptor modulators** (*Raloxifene*) |
| Vitamin D | vitamin D |
| s. Estrogene/Östrogene – estrogens | |
| Kalzium | calcium |

Probiotika (*Escherichia coli*) – Probiotics (*Escherichia coli*)

## Psychopharmaka – Psychopharmacologic drugs

| | |
|---|---|
| s. Antidepressiva – antidepressants | |
| **Neuroleptika**/Antipsychotika (*Haloperidol*) | **neuroleptic**/antipsychotic agents (*Haloperidol*) |
| **Sedativa/Beruhigungsmittel** | **sedatives/tranquilizers** |
| Antihistaminika (*Doxylamin*) | antihistamines (*Doxylamine*) |
| Phytotherapeutika (*Baldrianwurzel*) | phytotherapeutics (*Valerian root*) |
| **s. Anxiolytika – Anxiolytics** | |
| **Hypnotika**/»Schlafmittel« | **hyponotics**/«sleep-inducing drugs» |
| Benzodiazepine (*Diazepam*), welche auch sedativ wirken | Benzodiazepines (*Diazepam*), which also function as tranquilizers |
| Z-drugs (*Zolpidem*) | z-drugs (*Zolpidem*) |
| **Psychostimulzanien** (*Methylphenidat*) | **central nervous system stimulants** (*Methylphenidate*) |
| **Stimmungsstabilisierer** (*Lithium*) | **mood stabilizers** (*Lithium*) |
| **Psychotomimetika/Halluzinogene** (*Psilocin*), der Vollständigkeit aufgeführt | **psychodysleptics** (*Psilocin*), listed for the sake of completeness |

## Schilddrüsentherapie – Thyroid therapy

| Jodid | Iodide |
|---|---|
| **Schilddrüsenhormone** (*Levothyroxin*) | **thyroid hormones** (*Levothyroxine*) |
| **Thyreostatika** (*Thiamazol*) | **thyrostatics** (*Thiamazole*) |

Steroidhormone – Steroid hormones (s. Hormone – hormones)

Spasmolytika (*Butylscopolamin*) – Antispasmodics (*Butylscopolamine*)

## Virustatika – Antivirals

| | |
|---|---|
| Entry-Inhibitoren/Fusionsinhibitoren (*Maraviroc*) | entry-inhibitors/fusion inhibitors (*Maraviroc*) |
| Hemmstoff des viralen Uncoating (*Amantadin*) | viral uncoating inhibitors (*Amantadine*) |
| Integraseinhibitoren (INI) (*Raltegravir*) | integrase inhibitors (INI) (*Raltegravir*) |
| Neuraminidase-Hemmer (*Oseltamivir*) | neuraminidase inhibitors (*Oseltamivir*) |
| **Polymeraseinhibitoren** | **polymerase inhibitors** |
| Nucleosidanaloga (*Aciclovir*) | nucleoside analogues (*Aciclovir*) |
| Nucleotidanaloga (*Adefovir*) | nucleotide analogues (*Adefovir*) |
| nicht-nucleosidische Inhibitoren (*Dasabuvir*) | non-nucleoside inhibitors (*Dasabuvir*) |
| Proteaseinhibitoren (PI) (*Lopinavir*) | protease inhibitors (*Lopinavir*) |
| **Reverse-Transkriptase-Inhibitoren** | **reverse transcriptase inhibitors** |
| Nucleosidische Reverse-Transkriptase-Inhibitoren (NRTI) (*Zidovudin*) | nucleoside reverse transcriptase inhibitors (NRTI) (*Zidovudine*) |
| Nucleotidanaloge Reverse-Transkriptase-Inhibitoren (NtRTI) (*Tenofovir*) | nucleotide (analogue) reverse transcriptase inhibitors (NtRTI) (*Tenofovir*) |
| nicht-nucleosidische Reverse-Transkriptase-Inhibitoren (NNRTI) (*Doravirin*) | non-nucleoside reverse transcriptase inhibitor (*Doravirine*) |

## Vitamine – Vitamins

| | |
|---|---|
| *Vitamin A/Retinol* | *Vitamin A/Retinol* |
| *Vitamin $B_1$/Thiamin* | *Vitamin $B_1$/Thiamine* |
| *Vitamin $B_2$/Riboflavin* | *Vitamin $B_2$/Riboflavin* |
| *Vitamin $B_3$/Niacin/Nicotinsäure* | *Vitamin $B_3$/niacin/nicotinic acid* |
| *Vitamin $B_5$/Pantothensäure* | *Vitamin $B_5$/pantothenic acid* |

I Basiswissen – Basic Knowledge

| | |
|---|---|
| Vitamin $B_6$/Pyridoxin | Vitamin $B_6$/Pyridoxine |
| Vitamin $B_{12}$/Cobalamin | Vitamin $B_{12}$/Cobalamin |
| Vitamin C/Ascorbinsäure | Vitamin C/Ascorbic acid |
| Vitamin D/Calciferol | Vitamin D/Calciferol |
| Vitamin E/Tocopherol | Vitamin E/Tocopherol |
| Vitamin H (Vitamin $B_7$)/Biotin | Vitamin H (Vitamin $B_7$)/Biotin |
| Vitamin K | Vitamin K |
| Folsäure (Vitamin $B_9$/Vitamin $B_{11}$/Vitamin M) | Folic acid (vitamin $B_9$/vitamin $B_{11}$/vitamin M) |
| Multivitaminprodukte | multivitamin products |
| Vitamin-Vorstufen (*Benfotiamin*) | vitamin precursors (*Benfotiamine*) |

Zytostatika – Cytostatics

| | |
|---|---|
| alkylierende Substanzen/Alkylanzien (*Cisplatin*) | alkylating drugs (*Cisplatin*) |
| **Mitosehemmstoffe** (*Vincristin*) | **mitotic inhibitors** (*Vincristine*) |
| **Topoisomerasehemmer** (*Irinotecan*) | **topoisomerase inhibitors** (*Irinotecan*) |
| **Folsäure-Antagonisten** (*Methotrexat*) | **folic acid antagonists** (*Methotrexate*) |
| **Antimetabolite** (*Mercaptopurin*) | **antimetabolites** (*Mercaptopurine*) |
| **Enzyme/Differenzierungsinduktoren** (*Asparaginase*) | **enzymes/differentiation inductors** (*Asparaginase*) |
| **Hormone/Anti-Hormone** (*Tamoxifen*) | **hormones/anti-hormones** (*Tamoxifen*) |
| **Aromatasehemmer** (*Anastrozol*) | **aromatase inhibitors** (*Anastrozole*) |
| zytostatische Antibiotika (*Doxorubicin*) | antibiotics with cytostatic activity (*Doxorubicin*) |
| zytostatische Antikörper (*Trastuzumab*) | antibodies with cytostatic activity (*Trastuzumab*) |
| **Proteinkinase-Inhibitoren** (*Erlotinib*) | **protein kinase inhibitors** (*Erlotinib*) |
| **Proteoasom-Inhibitoren** (*Bortezomib*) | **proteasome inhibitors** (*Bortezomib*) |
| *sonstige* z. B. Hydroxycarbamid (*Hydroxyharnstoff*) | *others* e. g. hydroxycarbamide (*Hydroxyurea*) |

> **Beispiel – example**
>
> *Amoxicillin belongs to the drug class of β-lactam antibiotics.*
> Amoxicillin gehört zur Wirkstoffklasse der ß-Laktam-Antibiotika.

# 3 Pharmakotherapie – Pharmacotherapy

## 3.1 Grundbegriffe – General expressions

In Kap. 3.1 sind allgemeine Begriffe und Formulierungen zu den unterschiedlichen Themenbereichen der Pharmakotherapie aufgelistet.

Within chapter 3.1 general terms and phrases concerning pharmacotherapy-related subject areas are listed.

### 3.1.1 Produkttyp – Product type

| | |
|---|---|
| Arzneimittel | medicine/drug/medicinal product |
| verschreibungspflichtige Arzneimittel | prescription-only medicines (POM) |
| freiverkäufliche Arzneimittel<br>*Diese Arzneimittel sind in Deutschland auch außerhalb von Apotheken erhältlich.* | over-the-counter (OTC) medicines/general sales list medicines<br>*These medicines are also available outside of community pharmacies in Germany.* |
| apothekenpflichtige Arzneimittel<br>*Diese Arzneimittel sind in Deutschland nur in Apotheken erhältlich.* | over-the-counter (OTC) medicines/pharmacy-only medicines<br>*These medicines are only available in community pharmacies in Germany* |
| Betäubungsmittel | controlled substances/sometimes addictive opoids are labelled as »narcotics« |
| Tierarzneimittel | veterinary medicine |
| Blutprodukt(e) | blood product(s) |
| Hilfsmittel | therapeutic appliance(s) |
| Homöopathikum/Homöopathika | Homeopathic(s) |
| komplementärmedizinische Produkte und alternative Produkte | complementary and alternative medicines (CAM) |
| Kosmetikum/Kosmetika | cosmetic(s) |
| Medizinprodukt(e) | medical device(s) |
| Nahrungsergänzungsmittel | nutritional supplements |

## 3.1.2 Arzneimittelinformation – Drug information

| | |
|---|---|
| Fachinformation | drug label (AE)/summary of product characteristics (SmPC) (BE) |
| Beipackzettel/Gebrauchsinformation/ Packungsbeilage | product information leaflet (PIL)/package leaflet/patient information leaflet/package insert |
| Datenbank | database |

## 3.1.3 Pharmakotherapiebezogene Begriffe – Pharmacotherapy-related terms

| | |
|---|---|
| Adhärenz | adherence |
| Applikationshilfe | application aid |
| Arzneimittelabusus | drug misuse/drug abuse |
| arzneimittelbezogene Probleme (ABP) | drug-related problems (DRP) |
| Arzneimitteltherapiesicherheit (AMTS) | medication safety |
| Aufbewahrung von Arzneimitteln ▶ Kap. 3.5.5, Lagerungshinweise | storage of medication s. chapter 3.5.5, Storage information |
| die Beratung/beraten | the consultation/to counsel |
| Compliance | compliance |
| Dosierung/Dosis ▶ Kap. 3.5.2, Anwendungshinweise | dosage/dose s. chapter 3.5.2, Administration directions |
| die Dosierung anpassen | to adjust the dosage |
| gefälschtes Arzneimittel | counterfeit medicine |
| Indikation | indication |
| Kontraindikation | contraindication |
| Kunde | customer/client |
| (Medikamenten-)abhängigkeit | drug addiction/drug dependence |
| Medikamentenausweis (z. B. für den Zoll) | medication card (e. g. for customs)/pill card |
| Medikationsanalyse | medication review |
| eine Medikationsanalyse durchführen | to conduct a medication review |
| Medikationsfehler | medication error |
| Medikationsplan | medication plan/medication schedule/ treatment plan |
| Monitoring | monitoring |

| | |
|---|---|
| Monotherapie | monotherapy |
| Kombinationstherapie | combination therapy |
| Nebenwirkung(en) ▶ Kap. 3.5.3, Nebenwirkungen | side effect(s) s. chapter 3.5.3, Side effects |
| Off-label-Use | off-label use |
| Patientensicherheit | patient safety |
| Patient | patient |
| Pharmakovigilanz | pharmacovigilance |
| Polypharmazie | polypharmacy |
| Qualität | quality |
| Rezept ▶ Kap. 4.5.1, Das Rezept | Prescription s. chapter 4.5.1, The prescription |
| Schaden | harm/damage |
| Selbstmedikation | self-medication |
| Selbstversorgung/Selbstmedikation (inkl. nicht medikamentöser Maßnahmen) | self-care |
| therapeutische Breite | therapeutic margin |
| Theophyllin hat eine enge therapeutische Breite. | Theophylline has a narrow therapeutic margin. |
| Therapieabbruch/eine Therapie abbrechen | therapy termination/to discontinue a therapy |
| Toleranz | tolerance |
| Unbedenklichkeit | harmlessness |
| Wechselwirkung(en)/Interaktion(en) ▶ Kap. 3.5.4 | interaction(s) s. chapter 3.5.4, Interactions |
| Wirksamkeit (unter Routinebedingungen ▶ Kap. 2.1, Grundlagen) | effectiveness (under routine conditions, s. chapter 2.1, Basics) |
| Zulassung | marketing authorisation/drug approval |

## 3.1.4 Patientengruppe – Patient group

| | |
|---|---|
| Erwachsene | adults |
| Heranwachsende/Teenager | adolescents (teenager) |
| Kinder | children |
| Kleinkind | infant/toddler |
| Baby/Säugling | baby/infant |

> **Beispiel – example**
>
> *Seawater nasal sprays are considered to be medical devices, because their effect is limited to a physical effect.*
> Meerwassernasensprays werden als Medizinprodukte aufgefasst, da ihre Wirkung auf einen physikalischen Effekt beschränkt ist.

## 3.2 Darreichungsform – Dosage form

Darreichungsformen werden oft nach dem Aggregatszustand oder der Anwendungsart klassifiziert. Untenstehend in Kap. 3.2 ist eine Einteilung nach Aggregatszustand zu sehen.

Dosage forms are often classified based on physical form or route of administration. In chapter 3.2 a classification based on the physical form is displayed.

Darreichungsform – Dosage form

| feste Zubereitungsformen | solid dosage forms |
|---|---|
| Granulat | granule(s) |
| Kapsel | capsule |
| Puder (im Englischen erfolgt keine Unterscheidung zwischen Puder und Pulver) | powder |
| Pulver | powder |
| Tablette | tablet |
| **Subkategorien** | **subcategories** |
| Brausetablette | effervescent tablet |
| Hartkapsel (z. B. Hydroxypropylmethylcellulose (HPMC)-Kapsel) | hard-(XY (shell material e. g. hydroxypropyl methylcellulose) capsule |
| Weichkapsel (z. B. Weichgelatinekapsel) | soft-(XY (shell material e. g. gelatine))-capsule |
| Kautablette | chewable tablet |
| Lutschtablette | lozenge |
| Pastille(n) | pastille(s) |
| Wundpuder/Talkpuder | dusting powder |

| flüssige Zubereitungsformen | liquid dosage forms |
|---|---|
| Emulsion | emulsion |
| Infusion | infusion |
| Injektion | injection |
| Lösung | solution |
| Suspension | suspension |
| **Subkategorien** | **subcategories** |
| Gurgelwasser | gargle |
| Hustensaft/-sirup | linctus/coughing syrup |
| Einlauf/Klistier/Klysma | enema |
| Augentropfen | eye drops |
| Mundspülung | mouthwash |
| Nasenspray | nasal spray |
| Nasentropfen | nasal drops |
| Ohrentropfen | ear drops |
| Spülung | douche/rinse |
| Tropfen | drops |

| halbfeste Zubereitungsformen | semi-solid dosage forms |
|---|---|
| Creme | cream |
| Gel | gel |
| Lotion | lotion |
| Paste | paste |
| Salbe | ointment/salve |
| Zäpfchen | suppository |
| **Subkategorien** | **subcategories** |
| Augensalbe | opthalmic ointment |
| Liniment/Einreibemittel | liniment |
| Pessar/Vaginalzäpfchen | pessary/vaginal suppository |
| Pflaster (Haut-/transdermales, auch als umgangssprachliches Synonym für Wundschnellverband verwendet) | plaster/patch sometimes labelled as bandage (skin/transdermal) |
| Schaum | foam |
| Shampoo | shampoo |

| Subkategorien | subcategories |
|---|---|
| Umschlag/Maske/Wickel | poultice |
| Vaginalkapseln | vaginal capsules |
| Vaginalring | vaginal ring |
| Vaginaltabletten | compressed pessaries/vaginal tablet |
| **Inhalatoren – inhalers** | |
| Pulverinhalatoren | dry-powder inhalers |
| Dosieraerosol-Inhalatoren | (pressurized) metered-dose aerosol inhalers |
| Vernebler (z. B. *PARI BOY®*) | nebulizer (AE)/nebuliser (BE) (e. g. *PARI BOY®*) |
| Inhalationshilfe (spacer) | holding chamber (spacer) |

**Beispiel – example**

*Y: This is a dry-powder inhaler. Are you familiar with its usage? In case you want to reread the instructions you can have a look at point 3 on the package leaflet.*
S: Das ist ein Pulverinhalator. Sind Sie mit der Anwendung vertraut? Für den Fall, dass Sie die Anleitung nochmal lesen möchten, finden Sie die Anwendung unter Punkt 3 im Beipackzettel beschrieben.

## 3.3  Aggregatzustand – Physical form

Aggregatszustand – State of aggregation

| fest | solid |
|---|---|
| flüssig | liquid |
| gasförmig | gaseous |

**Beispiel – example**

gasförmiger Stickstoff – *gaseous nitrogen*

3 Pharmakotherapie – Pharmacotherapy

## 3.4 Arzneistoffformulierung – Drug formulation

In Kap. 3.4 sind einige Begriffe und Beispiele zur Wirkstoffformulierung aufgelistet, die auch im Rahmen der Beratung in der Apotheke relevant sein können.

In chapter 3.4 drug formulation-related terms and examples terms regarding drug formulations are listed, that may also be relevant when counseling customers.

| Wirkstofffreisetzung | drug release |
|---|---|
| schnell einsetzende Wirkstofffreisetzung | immediate drug release |
| verzögerte Wirkstofffreisetzung | delayed drug release |
| magensaftresistente Tabletten (z. B.) | enteric coated tablets (e. g.) |
| hinhaltende Freisetzung | sustained/prolonged/extended drug release |
| Retardtabletten (z. B.) | sustained release tablets/prolonged release tablets/extended release tablets/ »long-acting tablets« (e. g.) |
| veränderte Wirkstofffreisetzung | modified drug release |

| Tabletten-/Kapselüberzüge | tablet/capsule coats/coating |
|---|---|
| Filmüberzug | film coat |
| Zuckerüberzug/Dragee | sugar coat |

| allgemeine Begriffe | general terms |
|---|---|
| die vorzeitige Wirkstofffreisetzung vermeiden | to prevent premature drug release in the stomach |
| Gelatine | gelatine |
| Geschmacksmaskierung | taste masking |
| Hilfsstoffe | additives |
| Magenreizung vermeiden | to avoid gastric irritation |
| pH-abhängige Löslichkeit | pH-dependent solubility |
| säurelabil | acid-labil |
| Stabilität | stability |
| Überzug-Formulierung | coating formulation |
| wasserunlöslich | water insoluable |

**Beispiel – example**

*Y: This is an enteric coated capsule. The coat prevents premature drug release in the stomach and therefore gastric irritation.*
S: Das ist eine magensaftresistente Kapsel. Der Überzug verhindert die vorzeitige Wirkstofffreisetzung im Magen und daher auch eine Magenreizung.

## 3.5 Anwendung – Administration

In der untenstehenden Tabelle finden Sie Begriffe zu den Anwendungsarten und üblichen Abkürzungen.

You will find routes of administration within the table below and corresponding commonly used abbreviations.

### 3.5.1 Applikations-/Anwendungssart – Route of administration

Anwendungsart – Type of application

| | |
|---|---|
| aurikular (zum Ohr) | otic |
| bukkal (zur Backe/Wange) | buccal |
| dermal | dermal |
| inhalativ | inhaled/inhalation (inhal) |
| Einträufelung | instillation (instill) |
| intramuskulär | intramuscular |
| intravenös | intravenous |
| Implantat/implantieren | implant/to implant |
| nasal | nasal* (N) |
| opthalmisch/okular (zum Auge) | ophthalmic |
| parenteral (unter Umgehung des Darmes) | parenteral |
| peroral (p. o.)/oral | peroral/oral (O) |
| rektal | rectal |
| subkutan | subcutaneous |
| sublingual | sublingual (SL) |

## 3 Pharmakotherapie – Pharmacotherapy

| topisch | topical |
|---|---|
| transdermal | transdermal (TD) |
| (Tablette) zum Auflösen | (tablet) to be dissolved |
| vaginal | vaginal (V) |

\* bei der Verwendung des Adjektivs mit einem Verb wird im Englischen meist ein –ly beigefügt (z. B. to apply the drops nasally).

> **Beispiel – example**
>
> *Y: This is a sublingual tablet. In case of need place one underneath your tongue. The active ingredient will be resorbed rapidly and you will notice a relief within 30 seconds.*
> S: Das ist eine Sublingual-Tablette. Bei Bedarf sollten Sie eine Tablette unter der Zunge platzieren. Der Wirkstoff wird schnell resorbiert und Sie werden eine Linderung innerhalb von 30 Sekunden spüren.

### 3.5.2 Anwendungshinweise – Administration directions

In den untenstehenden Tabellen finden Sie sämtliche Anwendungshinweise, die Sie ihren Kunden mitgeben können oder müssen.

You will find various directions that you can or have to give your customer within the tables below.

Hinweise – Directions

| Art der Anwendung | type of administration |
|---|---|
| Sie sollten/sollen/müssen | you need to/should/must |
| etw. applizieren ((formal) (z. B. Augentropfen)) | to administer sth. (e. g. eye drops) |
| etw. aufkleben | to attach sth. |
| etw. auflösen | to dissolve sth. |
| etw. auftragen/anbringen | to apply sth. |
| etw. auswaschen | to rinse sth. |
| etw. behandeln | to treat sth. |
| etw. einführen | to insert sth. |
| etw. (ein-)nehmen | to take sth. |
| etw. einträufeln | to instill sth. |

| Art der Anwendung | type of administration |
|---|---|
| mit etw. gurgeln | to gargle with sth. |
| etw. herunterschlucken | to swallow sth. |
| etw. injizieren | to inject sth. |
| etw. kauen | to chew sth. |
| etw. lutschen | to suck sth. |
| etw. platzieren | to place sth. |
| etw. reduzieren | to reduce sth. |
| etw. trinken | to drink sth. |

| Anzahl der Einnahmen | number of applications |
|---|---|
| einmal | once |
| zweimal | twice |
| XY (hier die gewünschte Zahl einfügen)-mal | XY (insert number here) times |
| die Hälfte von XY | one/a half of XY |
| ein Drittel | one/a third |
| ein Viertel | one/a quarter |
| ein Fünftel | one/a fifth |
| pro Tag/täglich | per day/daily |
| pro Woche/wöchentlich | per week/weekly |
| pro Monat/monatlich | per month/monthly |
| pro Jahr/jährlich | per year/annually |

| Zeitpunkt der Einnahme | intake time |
|---|---|
| nüchtern | on an empty stomach/sober |
| zur Mahlzeit | with a meal |
| nach der Mahlzeit/postprandial | after a meal/postprandial |
| morgens | in the morning |
| mittags | in the afternoon |
| abends | in the evening |
| zur Nacht | at night |

## 3 Pharmakotherapie – Pharmacotherapy

| Dosierung | dosage |
|---|---|
| Dosisanpassung | dose adjustment |
| etw. ausschleichen/ausschleichend dosieren | to reduce/discontinue (a medication) gradually |
| etw. einschleichend dosieren | to gradually increase in dosage |
| Standarddosis | standard dose |
| Dosieranweisung | dosing instructions |
| dosisabhängige Faktoren | dose-dependent factors |
| Alter | age |
| Gewicht | weight |
| Leberfunktion | liver/hepatic function |
| Nierenfunktion | kidney/renal function |
| Begleiterkrankung/Komorbidität | comorbidity |
| (Ko-)Medikation | (co-)medication |
| Gramm (g) | gram (g)/gramme (BE) |
| Milligramm (mg) | milligram/milligramme (BE) |
| bis zu (z. B. 3-mal täglich) | up to (e. g. 3 times per day) |
| Maximaldosis | maximum dose |
| innerhalb von (z. B. 24 Stunden) | within (e. g. 24 hours) |
| Nehmen Sie nur XY, wenn XY auftritt. | Take XY only when XY occurs. |
| Sie können bis zu 3 Tabletten täglich einnehmen. | You can take up to 3 tablets per day. |
| Probieren Sie es erst einmal mit XY mg (oder z. B. einer Tablette). | Try taking XY mg (or e. g. one tablet) first. |
| Sollten sich die Symptome nicht verbessern, können Sie eine weitere Tablette einnehmen. | In case symptoms do not improve, you can take another tablet. |
| Bitte nehmen Sie nicht mehr als XY mg ein. | Please do not exceed taking XY mg. |
| Sie sollten die Creme 3-mal täglich 1 Monat lang anwenden. | You should apply the cream 3 times daily for 1 month. |

| besondere Hinweise | specific instructions |
|---|---|
| als Ganzes schlucken | to swallow as a whole |
| Bruchkerbe | score line |
| eine Tablette teilen | to divide a tablet/split |

I  Basiswissen – Basic Knowledge

| besondere Hinweise | specific instructions |
|---|---|
| etw. nicht zerbrechen/zerkleinern | do not crush sth. |
| etw. vermeiden (wenn Sie XY einnehmen) | to avoid sth. (when taking XY) |
| die gleichzeitige Einnahme von XY | the simultaneous intake of XY |
| Lagerhinweise ▶ Kap. 3.5.5, Lagerungshinweise | storage information s. chapter 3.5.5, Storage information |
| Tablettenteiler | tablet cutter/splitter |
| Wechselwirkungen ▶ Kap. 3.5.4, Wechselwirkungen | interactions s. chapter 3.5.4, Interactions |

**Beispiel – example**

Y: *Please shake the insulin gently before injecting it into an abdominal crease within 15 minutes before or immediately after a meal.*
S: *Bitte schütteln Sie das Insulin sanft, bevor Sie es innerhalb von 15 Minuten vor oder unmittelbar nach der Mahlzeit in eine Bauchfalte injizieren.*

### 3.5.3 Nebenwirkungen – Side effects

In den untenstehenden Tabellen sind Begriffe rund um das Thema Nebenwirkungen aufgelistet aufgeführt. Begriffe für Nebenwirkungen können auch aus ▶ Kap. 1.4 »Symptome« entnommen werden.

Within the tables below terms regarding side effects are being listed. Terms for side effects can also be found in the chapter 1.4 symptoms.

Nebenwirkungen – Side effects

| Definitionen | definitions |
|---|---|
| Nebenwirkung*/unerwünschte Arzneimittelwirkung (UAW) | side effect*/adverse reaction/adverse drug reaction (ADR)/adverse effect, suspected adverse reaction/undesirable effect |
| unerwünschtes Arzneimittelereignis (UAE))/unerwünschtes Ereignis | adverse event/adverse drug event (ADE)/ adverse experience |

| allgemeine Begriffe | general terms |
|---|---|
| Medikationsfehler | medication error |
| Off-label-Use | off-label use |
| Überdosierung | overdose |
| Potenzielle Nebenwirkungen umfassen XY | potential side effects include XY |

## 3 Pharmakotherapie – Pharmacotherapy

| allgemeine Begriffe | general terms |
|---|---|
| vorhersehbar | predictable |
| dosisabhängig | dose-related |
| Arzneimittelabusus/Arzneimittelmissbrauch | medicine/drug abuse |
| ungewollt | unwanted |
| etw. überdosieren | to overdose sth. |
| berufliche Exposition | occupational exposure |
| gelegentlich | occasional |
| gleichzeitig/simultan | at the same time/simultaniously |
| unerwünscht | undesirable |
| Effekt/Wirkung | effect |
| Beziehung | relationship |
| (mit einem Arzneimittel) verbunden sein | to be related to (a drug) |
| schädlich//toxisch | noxious/toxic |

| Art der Nebenwirkung | types of side effects/adverse reactions |
|---|---|
| dosisabhängig | dose-related/augmented |
| bizarr | bizarre |
| chronisch | chronic |
| verzögert | delayed |
| allergisch | allergic |
| idiosynkratisch | idiosyncratic |

| Schweregrad der Nebenwirkungen | severity of side effects |
|---|---|
| mild | mild |
| moderat | moderate |
| schwer | severe |
| lebensbedrohlich | life-threatening |
| tödlich/Tod | fatal/death |

| Häufigkeit der Nebenwirkung | frequency of side effects |
|---|---|
| sehr häufig (≥ 1/10, 1 Fall pro 10 Behandelten) | very common (≥ 1/10, 1 case per 10 treated patients) |
| häufig (< 1/10; ≥ 1/100) | common |

| Häufigkeit der Nebenwirkung | frequency of side effects |
|---|---|
| gelegentlich (< 1/100; ≥ 1/1.000) | uncommon |
| selten (< 1/1.000; ≥ 1/10.000) | rare |
| sehr selten (< 1/10.000) | very rare |
| unbekannt | unknown |

| Nebenwirkungen – Beispiele | side effects – examples |
|---|---|
| anticholinerger Effekt | anticholinergic effect |
| (Angio-) Ödem | (angio-) edema |
| (veränderter) pH-Wert | (change in the) pH-value |
| Agranulozytose | agranulocytosis |
| Allergie | allergy |
| allergische Reaktion | allergic reaction |
| Anaphylaxie | anaphylaxis |
| Arrhythmie | arrhythmia |
| Austrocknung (der Haut) | drying out (of the skin)/dehydration |
| Bluthochdruck/Hypertonie | hypertension/high blood pressure |
| Blutspiegelveränderung(en) | change in blood level(s) (of) |
| Blutungsneigung | bleeding tendency |
| Cushing-Syndrom | Cushing's syndrome |
| Darmträgheit | constipation/lethargy of the bowel |
| Diarrhö/Durchfall | diarrhea (AE)/diarrhoea (BE) |
| Dunkelfärbung des Stuhles | dark stools |
| Dyspepsie | dyspepsia |
| Exanthem | exanthema |
| gastrointestinale Beschwerden | gastrointestinal complaints |
| Gewichtsverlust | weight loss |
| Gewichtszunahme | weight gain |
| hepatotoxisch | hepatotoxic |
| Herzinsuffizienz | heart failure |
| Hirsutismus | hirsutism |
| Hyperkalziämie | hypercalcemia (AE)/hypercalcaemia (BE) |
| Hyperkaliämie | hyperkalemia (AE)/hyperkalaemia (BE) |

| Nebenwirkungen – Beispiele | side effects – examples |
|---|---|
| Hypernatriämie | hypernatremia (AE)/hypernatraemia (BE) |
| Hypersensitivität | hypersensivity |
| Hypokaliämie | hypokalemia (AE)/hypokalaemia (BE) |
| Hyponatriämie | hyponatremia (AE)/hyponatraemia (BE) |
| jucken/Utikaria | itching/urticaria |
| Lichtempfindlichkeit/Photosensitivität | photosensitivity |
| Magenbeschwerden | upset stomach/irritated stomach/stomach complaints |
| Müdigkeit | tiredness |
| Mundtrockenheit | dry mouth |
| nephrotoxisch | nephrotoxic |
| niedriger Blutdruck/Hypotonie | hypotension/low blood pressure |
| QT-Zeit-Verlängerung | QT-prolongation/prolonged QT interval |
| Rhabdomyolyse | rhabdomyolysis |
| schleimhautreizend | mucosa irritant/irritating to the mucosa |
| Schwindel | dizziness |
| Serotonin-Syndrom | serotonin syndrome |
| Stevens-Johnson-Syndrom | Stevens-Johnson-syndrome |
| teratogen | teratogenic |
| Verschlimmerung/Auslösen eines Asthma-Anfalles | asthma exacerbation |

\* Für den Begriff Nebenwirkung existieren im Deutschen und im Englischen Synonyme. Ähnlich klingende Begriffe werden fälschlicherweise in der Praxis oft verwechselt. Die Terminologie kann zudem auch je nach Land und zuständiger Arzneimittelbehörde variieren. Für die Beratung eines Kunden ist die Verwendung der Begriffe Nebenwirkung beziehungsweise side effect ausreichend.[7]

Several synonyms exist in German and English for the term side effect. Similarly sounding terms are sometimes used wrongly. The terminology can also vary across countries and drug authorities. Using the term side effect or Nebenwirkung respectively, is sufficient when counseling a customer.

---

7   European Medicines Agency (EMA): Guideline on good pharmacovigilance practices (GVP) – Annex I – Definitions (Rev 4). Stand: 09.10.2017. ;https://www.ema.europa.eu/en/documents/scientific-guideline/guideline-good-pharmacovigilance-practices-annex-i-definitions-rev-4_en.pdf [Abgerufen am 05.01.2022].
Finding and Learning about Side Effects (adverse reactions). Stand 05.10.2021. https://www.fda.gov/drugs/information-consumers-and-patients-drugs/finding-and-learning-about-side-effects-adverse-reactions [Abgerufen am 05.01.2022].

### Beispiel – example

Y: The doctor has prescribed a penicillin called Amoxicillin for you. Potential side effects include diarrhea, nausea or skin rashes. In case these occur, please discontinue to take Amoxicillin.
S: Der Arzt hat Ihnen ein Penicillin verschrieben. Potenzielle Nebenwirkungen umfassen Durchfall, Übelkeit oder Hautausschläge. Sollten diese auftreten, dann brechen Sie bitte die Einnahme von Amoxicillin ab.

## 3.5.4 Wechselwirkungen – Interactions

In den Tabellen sind Begriffe rund um das Thema Wechselwirkungen aufgeführt, die die Pharmakokinetik und Pharmakodynamik des Arzneistoffs betreffen könnten.

Within the tables below interaction-related terms are listed, that impact the drug's pharmacokinetic or pharmacodynamic properties.

Wechselwirkungen – Interactions

| pharmakodynamische Wechselwirkungen | phamacodynamic interactions |
|---|---|
| Aktivität am gleichen/ähnlichen Ziel(-ort) | activity at same/similar target |
| größerer/additiver/synergistischer Effekt | greater/additive/synergistic effect |
| reduzierter/antagonistischer Effekt | decreased/antagonist effect |
| Wenn niedrig dosierte Acetylsalicysäure (ASS) und Ibuprofen zusammen appliziert werden, kommt es zu einer Abnahme der Thrombozytenaggregationshemmung. | When a low dose Acetylicsalicylic acid (ASA) and Ibuprofen are applied together, there will be decrease in platelet aggregation inhibition. |
| pharmakokinetische Wechselwirkungen | pharmacokinetic interactions |
| gegenseitige Beeinflussung (von) | mutual influence (on) |
| Freisetzung | liberation |
| Absorption/Resorption | absorption |
| Verteilung | distribution |
| Plasmaproteinbindung | plasma protein binding |
| Metabolismus/Verstoffwechslung | metabolism |
| etw. metabolisieren | to metabolize (AE)/metabolise (BE) sth. |
| Cytochrom-P450-Enzym (CYP) | cytochrome P450 enzyme (CYP) |
| Enzyminduktion | enzyme induction |
| Enzyminhibition | enzyme inhibition |

## 3 Pharmakotherapie – Pharmacotherapy

| pharmakokinetische Wechselwirkungen | pharmacokinetic interactions |
|---|---|
| kompetitiv | competitive |
| nicht-kompetitiv | non-competitive |
| reversibel | reversible |
| nicht-reversibel/irreversibel | non-reversible/irreversible |
| XY (z. B. *Clarithromycin*) ist ein CYP-3A4-Inhibitor. | XY (e. g. *Clarithromycin*) is a CYP 3A4 inhibitor. |
| Wenn Simvastatin und Clarithromycin gleichzeitig appliziert werden, wird es einen Anstieg der Simvastatin-Plasma-Konzentration geben. | When Simvastatin and Clarithromycin are administered simultaneously, there will be an increase in Simvastatin plasma concentration. |
| Eliminierung/Ausscheidung | elimination/excretion |
| **allgemeine Begriffe** | **general terms** |
| Bioverfügbarkeit | bioavailability |
| Blutspiegelveränderung(en) | change in blood level(s) (of) |
| Diffusion | diffusion |
| Eiweißbindung | protein binding |
| gleichzeitig/simultan | at the same time/simultaniously |
| Arzneistoffinteraktionen | drug – drug interactions |
| Arzneistoff-Krankheitswechselwirkungen | drug – disease interactions |
| Arzneistoff – Nahrungs-/Getränkwechselwirkungen | drug – food/beverage interactions |
| Wirksamkeit | effectiveness |
| Wirkung | effect |
| XY kombinieren | to combine XY |
| XY nicht mischen | do not mix XY |
| XY und XY nicht gleichzeitig nehmen | do not take XY and XY at the same time |

Produkte/Stoffe, die häufig Wechselwirkungen eingehen –
Common products/substances that often interact with medicines

| Grapefruitsaft | grapefruit juice |
|---|---|
| Ionen/Mineralstoffe (z. B. *Eisen, Magnesium*) | ions/minerals (e. g. *iron, magnesium*) |
| Johanniskraut | St. John's wort (herb) |
| Milch | milk |

| | |
|---|---|
| Milchprodukte | milk products |
| Milchprodukte/Milcherzeugnisse | dairy products |
| Zigaretten(rauch) | cigarettes (cigarette smoke) |

**Beispiel – example**

*Y: The doctor has prescribed an antibiotic for you. Take 3 tablets per day, every 8 hours. Swallow the tablet with a glass of water, 1 hour before or 2 hours after each meal in an upright position. Do not take it with milk products, nor certain supplements such as Magnesium or Iron in order to avoid interactions.*
*S: Der Arzt hat Ihnen ein Antibiotikum verschrieben. Nehmen Sie 3 Tabletten täglich, alle 8 Stunden. Schlucken Sie die Tablette mit einem Glas Wasser 1 Stunde vor oder 2 Stunden nach der Mahlzeit in einer aufrechten Position. Nehmen Sie die Tabletten nicht zusammen mit Milchprodukten oder bestimmten Nahrungsergänzungsmitteln wie Magnesium oder Eisen ein, um Wechselwirkungen zu vermeiden.*

## 3.5.5 Lagerungshinweise – Storage information

In den Tabellen sind Begriffe und Formulierungen zu Lagerungshinweisen aufgeführt.

Within the tables below you will find terms and phrases that are relevant for medicines storage.
Umrechnung/conversion:
0° Celsius = 32° Farenheit,
° Celsius = (° Farenheit – 32) × 5/9,
° Farenheit = ° Celsius × 1,8 +32

Lagerungshinweise – Storage information

| Temperaturen | temperatures |
|---|---|
| (Grad) Celsius/°C | (degrees) Celsius/°C |
| (Grad) Farenheit/°F | (degrees) Farenheit/°F |
| warm | warm |
| Raumtemperatur (15–25°C/59–77°F) | room temperature (15–25°C/59–77°F) |
| kalt/kühl (8–15°C/46–59°F) | cool (8–15°C/46–59°F) |
| Kühlschrank (2–8°C/35,6–46°F) | refrigerated (2–8°C/35,6–46°F) |
| tiefgekühlt (< -15°C/< 5°F) | freezing (< -15°C/< 5°F) |

| Klimazonen | climate zones |
|---|---|
| feucht | moist |
| gemäßigt | temperate |
| heiß | hot |
| mediterran | mediterranean |
| polar | polar |
| trocken | dry |
| tropisch | tropical |

| hilfreiche Begriffe | helpful terms |
|---|---|
| Aufbrauchfrist (Haltbarkeit nach Anbruch) | grace period |
| Haltbarkeit | shelf life (shelf lives pl.)/durability |
| Verfalldatum | expiry date/expiration date |
| abgelaufenes Arzneimittel | expired medicine |
| einfrieren | to freeze |
| empfindlich sein | to be sensitive |
| Feuchtigkeit | moisture/humidity |
| Gefrierschrank | freezer |
| konserviert | preserved/conserved |
| unkonserviert | unpreserved |
| Kühlkette | cold chain/refrigeration chain |
| Kühlschrank | refrigerator/fridge |
| Kühltasche | cooler bag/cooling bag |
| Lagerbedingungen | storing conditions |
| Licht | light |
| Pillenbox/Arzneimittelbox/Tablettenbox | pill case/medicine box/tablet storage box |
| Siegel | seal |
| Stabilität (chemisch/physikalisch/mikrobiell) | stability (chemical/physical/microbial) |
| Thermometer | thermometer |
| unter variierenden Bedingungen lagern | to store under varying conditions |

| Hinweise | directions |
|---|---|
| vor Kindern geschützt lagern/für Kinder unzugänglich aufbewahren/außerhalb der Reichweite von Kindern aufbewahren | Keep out of reach of children |
| vor Licht/Feuchtigkeit geschützt lagern | to protect from light/humidity |
| kühl lagern | to store in cool conditions/in a cool place |
| Bewahren Sie das Arzneimittel nicht dort auf, wo es Erschütterungen/Sonnenlicht/Hitze ausgesetzt sein könnte. | Do not store the medicine where it may be exposed to vibrations/sunlight/heat. |
| Bitte das Arzneimittel nicht nach Ablauf des Verfalldatums einnehmen. | Please do not take the medicine after the expiry date. |
| Das Arzneimittel bei 2–8 °C aufbewahren. | Store the medicine between 2–8 °C. |
| Das Produkt bleibt unter XY Bedingungen stabil. | This product will remain stable under XY conditions. |
| Vor Sonneneinstrahlung geschützt lagern. | Avoid exposure to sunlight. |
| Unterhalb von 25 Grad Celsius lagern. | Keep below 25 degrees Celcius. |

**Beispiel – example**

Y: *This antibody is very heat sensitive. The refrigeration chain must not be disrupted.*
S: Dieser Antikörper ist sehr wärmeempfindlich. Die Kühlkette darf nicht unterbrochen werden.

## 3.6  Phytotherapie – Phytotherapy

Kunden fragen häufig nach pflanzlichen Wirkstoffen oder Pflanzenbestandteilen in beispielsweise Tees. Daher sind in Kap. 3.6 Pflanzenteile und Arzneipflanzen aufgeführt. Da die Trivialnamen der Pflanzen weltweit häufig sehr verschieden sind, wurden zudem auch die lateinischen Namen aufgeführt.

Since Customers often ask for herbal active ingredients or plant parts for teas for instance, various terms related to plant parts and medicinal plants were included in the tables in chapter 3.6. Trivial plant names vary substantially worldwide. Therefore, latin plant names were also integrated.

## 3.6.1 Pflanzenteile/Zubereitungen – Plant parts/preparations

| | |
|---|---|
| Beeren | fruit |
| Blätter | leaves |
| Blüten | flower/blossom |
| Decoct | decoct |
| Extrakt | extract |
| Kraut/Kräuter | herb/s |
| Mazerat | macerate |
| Rinde | cortex/bark |
| Samen | seed |
| Wurzel | root |

**Beispiel – example**

Y: *This capsule contains highly concentrated ginger root extract. It works well against nausea and has no side effects.*
S: Diese Kapsel enthält hoch konzentrierten Ingwerwurzelextrakt. Dieser wirkt gut gegen die Übelkeit und hat keine Nebenwirkungen.

## 3.6.2 Tees/Kräuter – Teas/herbals

| Pflanzenname | plant name/generic name | Droge/Zubereitung | plant drug/plant product | lateinischer Name/latin name |
|---|---|---|---|---|
| Anis | anise | Anisfrucht | aniseed | Pimpinella anisum |
| Arnika | arnica | Arnikablüten | arnica flowers | Arnicae flos |
| Artischocke | artichoke | Artischockenblätter/Artischockenextrakt | artichoke leaves/artichoke extract | Cynara scolymus |
| Baldrian | valerian | Baldrianwurzel | valerian root | Valeriana officinalis |
| Bärentraube | bearberry | Bärentraubenblätter | bearberry leaves | Arctostaphylus uvae-ursi |
| Beinwell | comfrey | Beinwellkraut | comfrey herbs | Symphti herba |
| Birke | birch | Birkenblätter | birch leaves | Betula pendula |
| Brennnessel | stinging nettle | Brennnesselblätter | stinging nettle leaves | Urtica dioica |
| echtes Süßholz | licorice (AE)/liquorice (BE) | Süßholzwurzel | licorice root (AE)/liquorice root (BE) | Glycyrrhiza glabra |
| Eibisch | marshmallow | Eibischwurzel | marshmallow root | Althaea officinalis |
| Enzian | gentian | Enzianwurzel | gentian root | Gentiana lutea |
| Fenchel | fennel | Fenchelfrüchte (Foeniculi amari fructus/Foeniculi dulcis fructus) | fennel fruit | Foeniculum vulgare |
| Frauenmantel | lady's mantle | Frauenmantelkraut | lady's mantle herb | Alchemilla vulgaris |
| Goldrute | goldenrod | Goldrutenkraut | goldenrod herb | Solidago vigaurea |
| Hauhechel | restharrow | Hauhechelwurzel | restharrow root | Ononis spinosa |

## 3 Pharmakotherapie – Pharmacotherapy

| Pflanzenname | plant name/generic name | Droge/Zubereitung | plant drug/plant product | lateinischer Name/latin name |
|---|---|---|---|---|
| Heidelbeere | blueberry/bilberry/blaeberry | Heidelbeerfrucht (meist getrocknet) | blueberry fruit/bilberry (dried) | Vaccinium myrtillus |
| Holunder | elder | Holunderblüten/Holunderfrüchte | elderflower/elderberries | Sambucus nigra |
| Hopfen | hop | Hopfenzapfen | hop cone | Humulus lupulus |
| Isländisches Moos/Lichen islandicus | iceland moss/iceland lichen | Isländisches Moos/Lichen islandicus | iceland moss/iceland lichen | Cetraria islandica |
| Javanische Gelbwurz/Kurkuma | turmeric/curcuma | – | turmeric root | Curcuma xanthorrhiza |
| Johanniskraut | St. John's wort/amber | Johanniskraut | St. John's wort herb | Hypericum perforatum |
| Kamille | camomile/chamomile | Kamillenblüten | camomile flowers/chamomile flowers/blossom | Matricaria recutita |
| Kümmel | caraway | Kümmelfrucht | caraway seed | Carum carvi |
| Linde | linde/lime | Lindenblüten | linde flowers/blossom/lime tree flowers | Tilia cordata |
| Löwenzahn | dandelion | Löwenzahnkraut/-wurzel | dandelion herb/root | Taraxacum officinale |
| Mädesüß | meadowsweet | Mädesüßblüten/-kraut | meadowsweet flowers/herb | Filipendula ulmaria |
| Mariendistel | milk thistle | Mariendistelfrucht/-kraut | milk thistle fruit/herb | Silybum marianum |
| Melisse | lemon balm/melissa | Melissenblätter | lemon balm leaves | Melissa officinalis |
| Orthosiphon/Javatee | java tea | Orthosiphonblätter | orthosiphon leaves | Orthosiphon aristatus |
| Passionsblume | passion flower | Passionsblumenkraut | passion flower herb | Passiflora incarnata |
| Pfefferminze | peppermint/mint | Pfefferminzeblätter/Pfefferminzekraut | peppermint leaves/peppermint herb | Mentha X piperita |

| Pflanzenname | plant name/generic name | Droge/Zubereitung | plant drug/plant product | lateinischer Name/latin name |
|---|---|---|---|---|
| Primel/Schlüsselblume | primrose/cowslip | Primelwurzel/Primelblüten | primrose root/primrose flower | Primula veris |
| Riesengoldrute | tall goldenrod/giant goldenrod | Riesengoldrutenkraut | tall goldenrod herb/giant goldenrod herb | Solidago gigantea |
| Ringelblume | marigold | Ringelblumenblüten | marigold flowers | Calendulae flos. |
| Salbei | sage | Salbeiblätter | sage leaves | Salvia officinalis |
| Sand-Flohkraut | sand plantain | Flohsamenschalen | psyllium seed husks | Plantago indica/afra |
| Schafgarbe | yarrow | Schafgarbenkraut | yarrow herb | Achillea millefolium |
| Sennes | senna | Sennesblätter | senna leaves | Cassia angustifolia/Cassia senna |
| Spitzwegerich | ribwort/buckhorn plantain/narrow leaf plantain | Spitzwegerichkraut | ribwort herb/buckhorn plantain herb/narrow leaf plantain herb | Plantago lanceolata |
| Tausendgüldenkraut | common centaury | Tausendgüldenkraut | centaury herb | Centaurium erythraea |
| Thymian | thyme | Thymianblätter | thyme leaves | Thymus vulgaris |
| Teufelskralle | devil's claw | Teufelskrallenwurzel | devil's claw root | Harpahophyti radix |
| Tormentill/Blutwurz | bloodroot/yellow tormentil | Blutwurzwurzelstock/Tormentillwurzelstock | tormentilla root | Potentilla erecta |
| Weide (Purpurweide) | willow | Weidenrinde | willow bark | Salix purpurea/Salix daphnoides |
| Wermut | wormwood/absinth(e) | Wermutkraut | wormwood herb | Artemisia absinthium |

### Beispiel – example

C: *I have slight abdominal cramps since this morning. Is there a herbal tea that you can recommend?*
Y: *Yes. We have a herbal tea combination of fennel, anise and caraway that will help relieve the cramps.*

C: *Ich habe seit heute Morgen leichte Bauchkrämpfe. Gibt es einen Tee, den Sie mir empfehlen können?*
Y: *Ja. Wir haben eine Tee-Kombination aus Fenchel, Anis und Kümmel, die helfen wird, die Krämpfe zu lindern.*

## 3.7 Rezepturen – Pharmaceutical compounding

Nachfolgend sind wichtige Begriffe rund um das Thema Rezepturen aufgeführt, die je nach Land auch variieren können. Es sind nur die wichtigsten Begriffe für das Kundengespräch und die Herstellung aufgelistet.

Below you will find important terms regarding pharmaceutical compounding. These terms can vary in different countries. Only expressions that are relevant for consultations are listed below.

Rezepturen – Pharmaceutical compounding

| | |
|---|---|
| Aluminiumtube | aluminium/metal ointment tube |
| Becherglas | beaker |
| Braunglasflasche | amber glass bottle |
| Dies ist eine Rezeptur. Wir müssen prüfen, ob wir alle Bestandteile haben. | This is an extemporaneous medication. We will have to check if we have all the necessary components. |
| Dosierungsanweisung | dosage instruction |
| Eigenherstellung von Arzneimitteln/Rezepturen | (pharmaceutical) compounding |
| etw. herstellen (z. B. eine Creme) | to compound sth. (e. g. a cream) |
| Grundlage | formulation base/prescription base/base |
| Herstellungsdatum | date of manufacture |
| Inkompatibilität | incompatibility |

| | |
|---|---|
| Kanüle | cannula/needle |
| kortisonhaltig | contains cortisone |
| Kruke | cream jar/ointment jar |
| Kühl lagern | store in a cool place |
| Labor (Rezepturlabor) | (compounding) laboratory |
| Messbecher | measuring cup |
| Messzylinder | (scaled) graduated cylinder/measuring cylinder |
| Nach der Anwendung bitte die Hände waschen. | Please wash your hands after the application. |
| Nicht über XY °C lagern | Do not store at temperatures above XY °C |
| Nur zur äußerlichen Anwendung | For external use only |
| Pipette | dropper/pipette |
| Rezeptur (-arzneimittel) | extemporaneous product/extemporaneously-compounded medicine/preparation/ medication/magistral preparation |
| Sie können es am XY (z. B. Montag) abholen. | You can pick it up on XY (e. g. Monday). |
| Spatel | spatula |
| Spenderdose (z. B. *unguator* ®/*topitec*®) | jar (e. g. *unguator*® jar/*topitec*® jar/cream jar/ointment jar) |
| Spritze | syringe |
| Tropfeinsatz | dropper insert |
| Tropfflasche | dropper bottle |
| Verwendbarkeitsfrist/Haltbarkeitsdatum | expiry date |
| Waage | balance |
| Weithalsglas | wide-neck glass |
| Wir können die Creme für Sie herstellen | We can compound the cream for you |
| Wirkstoff | active ingredient |

### Beispiel – example

*Y: The doctor has prescribed a compounding medication for you. We have to check first whether we have all the necessary components. We can then compound the cortisone cream for you. You can pick it up on Monday.*
S: Der Arzt hat Ihnen ein Rezepturarzneimittel verschrieben. Wir müssen überprüfen, ob wir alle nötigen Komponenten haben. Wir können dann die Kortison-Creme für Sie herstellen. Sie können diese am Montag abholen.

## 3.8 Wundversorgung – Wound treatment

In der Tabelle unten ist eine Auswahl an Verbandstoffen und entsprechendem Zubehör aufgelistet.

Within the table below a selection of wound dressings and equipment is presented.

### 3.8.1 Verbandstoffe – Wound dressings

| | |
|---|---|
| Aktivkohle-Wundverband | charcoal dressing |
| Alginatverband | alginate dressing |
| Desinfektionsmittel | disinfectant/antiseptic |
| Gaze/Verbandmull/Gazevierecke | gauze/gauze squares |
| Hydrogelverband | hydrogel dressing |
| Hydrokolloidverband | hydrocolloid dressing |
| Idealbinde | elastic bandage/elastic conforming bandage |
| imprägniertes/beschichtetes Netz/Gitterauflage | impregnated/coated meshes (interfere dressings/low adherence dressings) |
| Klebestreifen/Haftstreifen | adhesive strips |
| kohäsive Bandage/Verband | self-adhering bandage |
| Mullkompresse | compression bandage/gauze dressing/gauze compress |
| Mundschutz | face mask/surgical mask/mouthguard |
| Netzverband | net bandage/elastic net bandage |
| Notverband | improvised bandage/first-aid dressing |
| Paraffingaze | paraffin gauze |
| Pflaster (umgangssprachlich) bzw. Wundschnellverband/ Pflaster (Haut-/transdermales) | plaster/patch (skin/transdermal) |
| Primärverband | primary dressing |
| Saugkompressen | absorbent dressing pad |
| Schaumverband | foam wound dressing |
| Schlauchverband | tube bandage/tubular elastic dressing |
| Sekundärverband/Zusatzverband | secondary dressing |
| selbstklebendes Klebeband/adhäsives Klebeband | adhesive tape roll |

| | |
|---|---|
| Silberverband | silver dressing |
| Tapeverband | tape bandage/tape |
| transparentes Klebeband | transparent film |
| Tupfer | gauze pad(s) |
| Verband/Verbände | dressing/bandage |
| Verbandmaterial | dressing material |
| Waschhandschuhe | washing gloves/wash cloths |
| Watte | absorbent cotton (AE)/cotton wool (BE) |
| Wundauflage | wound dressing/wound pad |
| Wundnahtstreifen | wound closure strips |
| Wundschnellverband/selbsthaftender Wundverband (umgangssprachlich: Pflaster) | s. plaster (bandage) |

### Beispiel – example

C: Hello. My father has accidentally cut himself while cooking. We need a wound dressing. Do you have small plasters?
K: Hallo. Mein Vater hat sich versehentlich beim Kochen geschnitten. Wir brauchen einen Wundverband. Haben Sie kleine Pflaster?

## 3.8.2 Wundarten – Types of wounds

| | |
|---|---|
| Hautabschürfung/Schürfwunde | abrasion |
| Penetration/Durchbohrung | penetration |
| Punktuation/Einstich | puncture |
| Riss-, Schnitt-, Kratzwunde | laceration |
| Ulkus/Geschwür | ulcer |
| Verbrennung/Brandwunde | burn |

### Beispiel – example

C: I touched the stove by mistake and burned my hands. There is even a blister on one of the hands. Do you think I should go and see a doctor?
K: Ich habe aus Versehen die Herdplatte angefasst und mir die Hände verbrannt. Auf einer Hand habe ich sogar eine Blase. Sollte ich einen Arzt aufsuchen?

# II    Die Beratung – The consultation

# 4 Beratungspraxis – Consultation practice

## 4.1 Die Begrüßung – The Greeting

Am Anfang eines jeden Gespräches findet die Begrüßung statt. In der Tabelle finden Sie einige Begrüßungsvorschläge.

The initial part of a conversation consists of a greeting. In the table you will find suggestions for a salutation.

Begrüßung – Greeting

| | |
|---|---|
| Guten Morgen | Good morning |
| Guten Tag | Good afternoon |
| Guten Abend | Good evening |
| Hallo | Hello |
| Hallo, wie geht es dir/Ihnen? | Hello, how are you?* |
| Hallo/Guten Tag | Good day (Australia) |
| Was kann ich für Sie tun? | What can I do for you? |
| Wie kann ich Ihnen helfen? | How can I help you? |
| Wie könnte ich Ihnen helfen? | How may I help you? |
| Hallo, Ich bin der Apotheker im Dienst. | Hello, I am the pharmacist on duty. (not commonly used in Germany) |

* Diese Floskel ist im amerikanischen Englisch sehr verbreitet. Sie wird als Begrüßungsfloskel verwendet. Es wird in der Regel mit »Good, thanks.« geantwortet. Diese Floskel zielt nicht darauf ab, Ihren Status Quo zu erfragen, sondern dient lediglich als Begrüßungsformel. Ihr Gegenüber erwartet also nicht eine ausführliche Beschreibung Ihres physischen und psychischen Zustandes.

> **Beispiel – example**
>
> Y: *Hello, what can I do for you?*
> S: Guten Tag, was kann ich für Sie tun?

## 4.2 Abschlussformeln und Fragen – Finishing phrases and questions

| | |
|---|---|
| Haben Sie noch Fragen? | Do you have any questions? |
| Gibt es noch etwas, was Sie besprechen möchten? | Is there anything else you would like to discuss? |
| Ich hoffe, das war hilfreich. | I hope that was helpful. |
| Ich hoffe, dass ich Ihnen helfen konnte. | I hope I was able to help you. |
| Viel Glück/Erfolg beim Finden von XY. | Good luck (in) finding XY. |
| Lassen Sie mich helfen, die Tür aufzumachen/aufzuhalten. | Let me help you by opening/holding the door. |
| Machen Sie es gut und haben Sie einen schönen Tag. | Take care and have a good day. |
| Ich hoffe, Sie werden sich bald besser fühlen/Gute Besserung. | I hope you will feel better soon/get well soon. |
| Auf Wiedersehen | Goodbye/Bye/Bye-bye |

**Beispiel – example**

Y: *Now here is 12.50 Euros in change. Take care and have a good day.*
*[In UK/US the decimal point is used to divide numbers rather than the (decimal) comma.]*
S: Hier sind 12,50 Euro Rückgeld. Machen Sie's gut und einen schönen Tag noch!
[Im Englischen (UK/US) wird ein Punkt anstelle eines Kommas verwendet, um Zahlen zu trennen.]

## 4.3 Wichtige Fragen und Begriffe – Important questions and terms

Genug Informationen über den Kunden und sein Anliegen bilden die Entscheidungsgrundlage in der Beratung. **Merkhilfen** können hilfreich sein, um sicherzugehen, dass die wichtigsten Aspekte abgefragt werden. Sie sind allerdings mit Vorsicht zu betrachten, da sie nicht immer alle Inhalte abdecken. Ein Beispiel anhand der WWHAM-Merkhilfe ist hier aufgeführt:

W – Who is the patient/Wer ist der Patient? (age, sex, pregnancy yes/no – Alter, Geschlecht, Schwangerschaft ja/nein)
W – What symptoms is the patient experiencing/Welche Symptome sind beim Patienten aufgetreten?
H – How long have the symptoms been present/Wie lange sind die Symptome vorhanden?
A – Action taken so far/Was wurde bisher unternommen?
M – Medication being taken/Werden Medikamente eingenommen?

Sufficient information form the basis for decision-making when it comes to counseling. Mnemonics can be useful for remembering what aspects need to be addressed. They need to be treated with caution however since they may not cover all necessary content. An example based on the WWHAM-mnemonic is displayed above.[8]

Hier finden Sie allgemeine Formulierungsvorschläge für Fragen und Empfehlungen sowie Apothekenspezifische Begriffe:
Here you will find general suggestions for formulating your questions and recommendations and Pharmacy-specific terms.

## Allgemeine Fragen/Begriffe in der Beratung – General counseling questions/expressions

| | |
|---|---|
| Was führt Sie heute zu uns (in die Apotheke)? | Hello, what brings you to the pharmacy today? |
| Ich würde Ihnen gerne ein paar Fragen stellen, um Ihnen besser weiterhelfen zu können. | I would like to ask you a few clarifying questions in order to help you better. |
| Ist das ok für Sie? | Is that alright with you? |
| Wie fühlen Sie sich? | How are you feeling? |
| Welche Symptome haben Sie/hast du? | What symptoms do you have?/What symptoms are you experiencing? |
| Wie würden Sie XY beschreiben? | How would you describe XY? |
| Wie fühlt sich XY an? | How does XY feel? |
| Auf einer Skala von 0 bis 10, die 10 beschreibt das Schlimmste, wie würden Sie XY bewerten? | On a scale from 0 to 10, whereas 10 is the worst, how would you rate XY? |
| Welcher Körperbereich ist betroffen? | What part of the body is affected? |

---

8  Blenkinsopp A, Paxton P, Blenkinsopp J (2009): Symptoms in the Pharmacy: A Guide to the Management of Common Illness, 6th Edition. Oxford.

## II Die Beratung – The consultation

| | |
|---|---|
| Wo ist XY (z. B. die Wunde)? | Where is XY (e. g. the wound)? |
| Wann fing XY an? | When did XY start? |
| Seit wann sind die Symptome aufgetreten? | Since when did the symptoms occur? |
| Wie oft tritt XY auf? | How often does XY appear/occur? |
| Wann tritt XY auf?/Sagen Sie mir wann XY auftritt. | When does XY occur?/Tell me when XY occurs. |
| Gibt es etwas, das XY (z. B. den Juckreiz) lindert? | Does anything relieve XY (e. g. the itch)? |
| Gibt es etwas, dass XY verschlimmert? | Does anything make XY worse? |
| Warum tritt XY auf? Was denken Sie? | Why do you think this is happening? |
| Haben Sie eine Vermutung warum XY auftritt? | Do you have a suspicion why XY occurs? |
| Wie beeinflusst XY ihr alltägliches Leben? | How does XY affect your everyday life? |
| Haben Sie es von einem Arzt untersuchen lassen? | Have you already had it checked-up by a medical doctor/physician (AE)/General Practitioner (GP)/medical doctor (BE)? |
| Was ist Ihnen bei XY aufgefallen? | What have you noticed about XY? |
| Gibt es etwas Spezielles, was Ihnen Sorgen bereitet? | Is there anything in particular that worries you? |
| Ist XY in Ihrer Familie bereits aufgetreten? | Has XY occured in your family history? |
| Was haben Sie bisher getan/unternommen? | What actions have been taken so far? |
| Haben Sie weitere Erkrankungen? | Do you have any further diseases? |
| Ich frage Sie, um sicherzugehen, dass XY für Sie auch geeignet ist. | I am asking you this, because I would like to make sure that XY is suitable for you |
| Nehmen Sie noch andere Medikamente oder Nahrungsergänzungsmittel ein? | Do you take any other forms of medication or nutritional supplements? |
| Sind Sie gerade schwanger? | Are you currently pregnant? |
| Stillen Sie zurzeit? | Are you currently breastfeeding/nursing? |
| Alternativ: Dieses Arzneimittel darf nur angewendet werden, sofern eine Schwangerschaft oder Stillzeit ausgeschlossen werden kann. | Alternatively: This medicine can only be used, in case one can exclude pregnancy or is not currently nursing. |
| Haben Sie noch weitere Fragen? | Do you have any further questions? |
| Diese(s) Arzneimittel/Tabletten/Pillen sind verschreibungspflichtig. | These medications/tablets/pills are only available on prescription. |

| die Empfehlung formulieren | formulating your advice |
|---|---|
| Basierend auf Ihrer Beschreibung von XY/der Symptome, empfehle ich XY. | Based on your description of XY/the symptoms, I recommend XY. |
| Laut Ihrer Beschreibung Ihrer Symptome würde ich Ihnen empfehlen, XY mit XY zu behandeln. | According to the description of your symptoms, I would advise you to treat XY with XY. |
| Es scheint, dass Sie sich XY (z. B. eine Erkältung) eingefangen haben. | It seems that you caught XY (e. g. a cold). |
| Zur Unterstützung von XY empfehle ich Ihnen XY. | To support XY, I recommend XY. |
| Wir haben XY auf Lager. Ich hole es Ihnen gerne. Ich bin gleich wieder da. | We have XY in stock. I am happy to get it for you. I will be back in just a few seconds. |
| Sollten sich die Symptome nicht innerhalb von XY bessern, dann wenden Sie sich bitte an einen Arzt. | In case the symptoms do not improve within XY, please go and see a physician (AE)/general practicioner (BE)/medical doctor. |
| Anwendungshinweise s. Kap. 3.5.2 | intake instructions s. chapter 3.5.2 |
| Bitte nehmen Sie XY nicht mehr. | Please stop taking XY. |
| XY könnte mit XY wechselwirken/interagieren. | XY may interact with XY. |
| entlasten/lindern | to alleviate/to relieve |
| Selbstmanagemenet einer Erkrankung | self-managment of a condition/to self-manage a condition |

| apothekenspezifische Begriffe | pharmacy-specific terms |
|---|---|
| Abholschein | collection voucher |
| Abstand halten | to keep a distance |
| Apotheken-Kette | pharmacy chain |
| Apotheker/-in | pharmacist/(dispensing) chemist |
| Arzneimittel abgeben | to dispense medicines/drugs |
| Arzneimittel abholen | to collect someone's medicine/to pick up someone's medicine |
| Arzneimittel-Engpass/Lieferengpass | shortage of medicines/supply shortage |
| Belieferung | delivery/supply |
| Botendienst | courier/delivery service |
| Datenschutzgesetz | data protection law |
| durchschnittlicher Großhandelspreis | average wholesale medicine price |

II Die Beratung – The consultation

| apothekenspezifische Begriffe | pharmacy-specific terms |
|---|---|
| etw. auf Lager haben | to have sth. in stock |
| etw. bestellen | to order sth. |
| Hygienemaßnahmen | hygiene measures/sanitary measures |
| Krankenhaus-Apotheke | hospital pharmacy |
| Mehrwertsteuerrückerstattung | (valued added tax) VAT refund |
| nicht lieferbar/außer Handel | out of stock/unavailable/withdrawn from/off the market |
| öffentliche Apotheke | community/retail pharmacy |
| Pflegeheim | nursing home |
| pharmazeutische Dienstleistung (z. B. Blutdruckmessung) | pharmaceutical service (e. g. blood pressure measurement) |
| Pharmazeutisch-Kaufmännische(r) Assistent/in | pharmaceutical clerk |
| Pharmazeutisch-Technischer Assistent | pharmacy technician |
| Pharmazeutisches Personal | pharmaceutical staff |
| Preisschild | price tag/price sticker |
| Privatsphäre | privacy |
| Tragen von Mund- und Nasenschutz | to wear a mouth and nose protection |
| Quittung | receipt |
| steuerfrei | tax free |
| Versandapotheke/online Versandhandels-Apotheken | mail order pharmacy/online mail order pharmacies |
| Versorgung | supply |

| einrichtungsbezogene Begriffe | furniture-related terms |
|---|---|
| Beratungsraum(-ecke) | consultation room/corner |
| Kasse/Kassierer | cash desk/checkout/cashier |
| Komissionierer | pharmacy robot |
| Regal | shelf |
| Schublade | drawer |
| Tresen | counter |

## Beispiel – example

Y: *Hello, what can I do for you?*
C: *Hello. I need Ibuprofen.*
Y: *For whom is the medication?*
C: *It is for myself. I am planning to go on a cruise and would just like to complete my medical travel kit.*

S: Hallo, was kann ich für Sie tun?
K: Hallo, Ich brauche Ibuprofen.
S: Für wen ist das Arzneimittel?
K: Es ist für mich. Ich plane auf eine Kreuzfahrt zu gehen und möchte nur gerne meine Reiseapotheke vervollständigen.

## 4.4 Selbstmedikation – Self-medication

In der Apotheke fragen Kunden häufig nach bestimmten Produkten, die sich manchmal nicht den Arzneistoffklassen zuordnen lassen. Eine Auswahl ist in der untenstehenden Tabelle zu sehen. Beispielprodukte sind in den Klammern genannt. Der Begriff self-care bedeutet so viel wie Selbstversorgung und schließt auch nicht-medikamentöse Maßnahmen wie zum Beispiel Inhalieren ein.

Community Pharmacy clients inquire about certain products, that do not necessarily belong to a drug class. A selection of those products is provided below. Example-products are listed within the brackets.

| sonstige/häufig genutzte Produkte | other/commonly used products |
|---|---|
| Adstringenzien (*Aluminiumsalze*) | astringents (*Aluminium salts*) |
| Antiseborrhoika (*Selensulfid*) | antiseborrhoeic agents (*Selenium sulfide*) |
| Antitussiva für eine detailllierter Einteilung ▶ Kap. 5.1.1, Husten | antitussives/cough suppressant(s) – s. chapter 5.1.1, cough for a more detailed description |
| ätherische Öle (*Lavendelöl*) | essential oils/ethereal oils (*Lavender oil*) |
| Aufbaunahrungen (*Fresubin®*) | nutritional supplements/«high-calorie oral supplements» (*Fresubin®*) |
| Auqaretika (*Goldrutenkraut*) | aquaretics (*Goldenrod herb*) |
| Binden | (menstrual/sanitary) pads |
| Diätetika | dietetics/dietary products |

II Die Beratung – The consultation

| sonstige/häufig genutzte Produkte | other/commonly used products |
|---|---|
| (Slip-)Einlagen | daily liners |
| Entschäumer (*Dimeticon*) | (medical) defoamers/anti-foaming agents (*Dimethicone*) |
| Erkältungsmittel | cold remedies |
| Flächendesinfektionsmittel (*Bacillol*®) | surface disinfectants (*Bacillol*®) |
| Händedesinfektionsmittel (*Sterillium*®) | hand disinfectants (*Sterillium*®) |
| Handschuhe (Baumwolle/Latex/latexfrei) | (cotton/latex/latexfree) gloves |
| Homöopathika (gehört zu keiner Wirkstoffklasse, sondern beschreibt eher ein Therapieprinzip) | homeopathics (they do not belong to any specific drug class, but they rather represent a therapy principle) |
| Hygieneartikel | toiletries/sanitary products/hygiene articles |
| Immunstimulanzien (*Echinacea purpurea*) | immunostimulants (*Echinacea purpurea*) |
| Insektensprays (*Piperonylbutoxid*) | insect spray/bug spray (*Piperonyl butoxide*) |
| Keratolytika (*Salicylsäure*) | keratolytics (*Salicylic acid*) |
| Kompressionsstrümpfe | compression stockings |
| Kontaktlinsenflüssigkeit (Desinfektion und Aufbewahrung) (*Lenscare*®) | contact lens solution (disinfecting/cleaning and storage) (*Lenscare*®) |
| Kosmetika | cosmetics |
| Lactase (*Lactrase*®) | lactase (*Lactrase*®) |
| »Läusemittel«/Pedikulozide (*Permethrin*) | antipediculotic(s) (agents)/lousicides (*Permethrin*) |
| Masken | masks |
| Medizinprodukte | medical devices/medical products |
| Mundspüllösungen | mouth rinses/mouth rinsing solutions |
| Nahrungsergänzungsmittel | nutritional/dietary supplement(s) |
| Narbenkosmetika (*Kelofibrase*®) | scar care products |
| Nicotinpflaster/-kaugummis | nicotine patches/gums |
| Ödemprotektiva (*Aescin*) | edema-protective agents (*Aescin*) |
| Repellentien (*Icaridin*) | repellents (*Icaridin/Picaridin*) |
| Schleimlöser | mucolytics |
| Schmerzmittel | painkillers |
| Sekretolytika | secretolytics |
| Sonnencreme (*Ladival*®) | sunscreen (*Ladival*®) |
| Tampons | tampons |

| sonstige/häufig genutzte Produkte | other/commonly used products |
|---|---|
| Tränenersatzflüssigkeit | tear substitutes |
| Venensalben/-cremes/-gele | varicose (vein) salves/creams/gels/ointments |
| Wärmesalben/-cremes (*Capsaicin*) | warming salves/creams/ointments |
| Warzenmittel | verruca/wart remedies |
| Wunddesinfektionsmittel (*Octenidin*) | skin disinfectants (*Octenidine*) |

**Beispiel – example**

C: *Hello, I need pads. Do you sell these?*
K: Hallo, ich benötige Binden. Verkaufen Sie diese?

## 4.4.1 Grenzen der Selbstmedikation – Self-medication limits

Dieses Kapitel enthält Formulierungshilfen für den Fall, dass die Grenze der Selbstmedikation erreicht ist bzw. Sie Ihren Kunden an einen Arzt verweisen müssen. Die Rolle des Apothekers und der gesetzliche Handlungsrahmen variiert weltweit stark. In anderen Ländern können Apotheker beispielsweise auch Rezepte ausstellen. Es kann also durchaus sein, dass Sie Ihrem Kunden erklären müssen, dass er für bestimmte Anliegen hierzulande zu einem Arzt gehen muss. Im Kapitel Symptome (▶ Kap. 1.4) und Krankheiten (▶ Kap. 1.3) finden Sie Begriffe für sogenannte red flags.

This chapter contains phrases and expressions in case the limits of self-medication have been reached or you need to refer a patient to a medical doctor. The role and legal framework of action among pharmacists varies worldwide. Pharmacists may for example issue prescriptions. Therefore, it may be necessary to explain to your client, that he or she needs to see a medical doctor for certain matters. Within the chapter 1.4 symptoms and 1.3 diseases you will find terms for the so-called red flags.

**Verweis an andere Gesundheitsprofessionen – Referral to other health professionals**

| Dafür ist eine spezielle Behandlung notwendig. | You need to receive a special treatment. |
|---|---|
| Das ist gesetzlich verboten. | This is prohibited by law. |
| Das kann der Arzt zum Beispiel mithilfe einer Blutuntersuchung herausfinden. | The medical doctor can find that out through a blood test for instance. |

| | |
|---|---|
| Das kann nur der Arzt feststellen. | Only a medical doctor can determine that (or diagnose that). |
| Das kann nur ein Arzt verschreiben. | Only a medical doctor is allowed to prescribe that. |
| Das muss untersucht werden. | This needs to be examined/analysed. |
| Das muss sich ein Arzt ansehen. | This has to be analysed/examined by a doctor. |
| Es tut mir leid, aber das darf ich nicht injizieren. | I am sorry, but I am not allowed to inject it. |
| Harnuntersuchung | urinalysis |
| Ich darf keine Diagnose stellen. | I am not allowed to make a diagnosis. |
| Ich empfehle Ihnen dringend, ins Krankenhaus zu gehen. | I urgently recommend you to go to a hospital. |
| Ich empfehle Ihnen, zum Arzt zu gehen. | I recommend you to go and see a medical doctor. |
| Ich rufe einen Rettungswagen. | I will call an ambulance. |
| Sie müssen ins Krankenhaus gehen. | You have to go to a hospital. |
| So etwas dürfen wir nicht tun. | We are not allowed to do this. |
| Weitere Untersuchungen sind notwendig. | Further examinations are needed. |
| Wir dürfen keine Wundversorgung machen. | We are not allowed to provide any wound treatment. |
| XY könnte auf XY hindeuten. | XY can indicate that you may have (a) XY. |
| Red flag(s) | red flag(s) |

**Beispiel – example**

*Y: I strongly recommend you to go and see a doctor. Your blood pressure is too high.*
*S: Ich empfehle Ihnen dringend, einen Arzt aufzusuchen. Ihr Bludruck ist zu hoch.*

## 4.5 (Rx) Verschreibungspflichtige Arzneimittel – Prescription only medicines (POMs)

In diesem Abschnitt finden Sie Tabellen mit Begriffen und Sätzen/Satzbausteinen für die Beratung und/oder Abgabe von verschreibungspflichtigen Arzneimitteln.

4 Beratungspraxis – Consultation

In this section you will find tables that contain expressions as well as phrases which are useful for the pharmaceutical consultation and dispense of prescription-only-medicines.

## 4.5.1 Das Rezept – The prescription

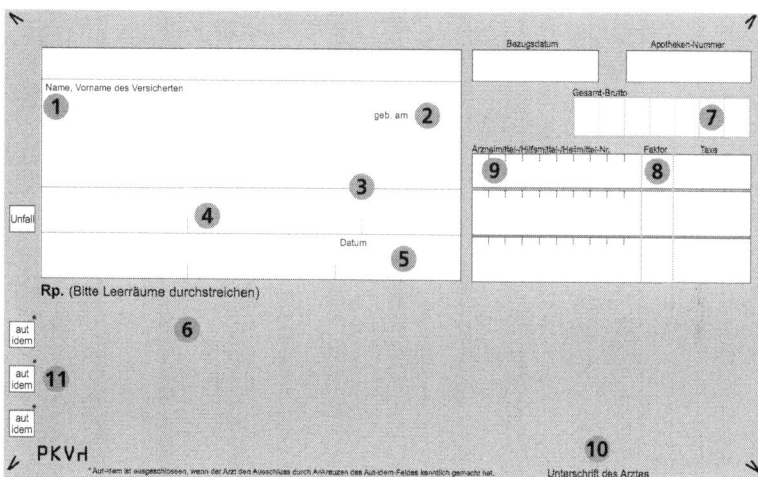

**1** patient's surname, name, address
– Nachname, Vorname des Patienten, Adresse

**2** date of birth
– Geburtsdatum

**3** (personal) identification number
– Personennummer

**4** insurance number
– Versicherungsnummer

**5** date of prescribing/date of issue
– Ausstellungsdatum

**6** medicine regimen
(name (usually brand name), strength, dose, dosage form administration, duration of intake, packaging size)
– Arzneimittelschema (Wirkstärke, Dosierung (Dosierplan), Darreichungsform, Einnahme (-hinweis), Dauer, Packungsgröße)

**7** gross price
– Bruttopreis

**8** factor/quantity
– Faktor/Menge

**9** pharmaceutical registration number (PZN)/appliance number
– Arzneimittel-/Hilfsmittelnummer

**10** name, registration number, signature of the prescriber
– Name, Registriernummer, Unterschrift des Verordners

**11** Nec Aut idem
– Do not substitute/dispense as written

Abb. 4.1: Angaben auf einem (Privat-)Rezept – private prescription details

87

## 4.5.2 Rx-Arzneimittel – Prescription only medicines

| Angaben auf dem Rezept | prescription details |
|---|---|
| Aut-Idem-Feld (auf Rezept) mit X versehen (»Nec Aut Idem«) | Do not substitute/dispense as written (*sinngemäße Übersetzung*) |
| Hilfsmittelnummer | appliance number |
| Datum | date |
| Zuzahlungsbefreiung | copayment-exempt |

| Rezeptarten (jeweilige Rezeptfarbe) | prescription types (prescription color in Germany) |
|---|---|
| Berufsgenossenschaftsrezept-(BG) Rezept (rosa) | employer's liability insurance association-prescription (pink) |
| Betäubungsmittelrezept (gelb) | controlled substance prescription (yellow) |
| Empfehlungsrezept/Arztempfehlung (grün) | (doctoral) recommendation/OTC-prescription (green) |
| Entlassrezept (nach stationärem Krankenhausaufenthalt, rosa) | discharge prescription (after an inpatient hospital stay, pink) |
| Hilfsmittelrezept (rosa) | therapeutic appliance prescription (pink) |
| Isotretioninrezept (für Frauen im gebärfähigen Alter, rosa) | Isotretion-prescription (for women of childbearing age, pink) |
| Kassenrezept (rosa) | panel prescription (pink) |
| Privatrezept (blau) | private prescription (blue) |
| T-Rezept (für Thalidomid, Lenalidomid, Pomalidomid, weiß) | T-prescription (used for the dispense of Thalidomide, Lenalidomide, Pomalidomide, white) |
| §-27a-Rezept (künstliche Befruchtung, rosa) | §-27a-prescription (artificial fertilization (AE)/fertilisation (BE)/insemination, pink) |
| elektronisches Rezept/E-Rezept | electronic prescription |

| Rx-bezogene Begriffe | Rx-related terms |
|---|---|
| Datenmatrix-Code | data matrix code |
| Rezeptanforderungen | prescription requirements |
| Rezeptgebühr | prescription charge |
| Akutversorgung | acute/immediate care |
| Änderung | amendment |
| Anweisung(en) (Dosierung) | directions/instructions |
| eine Genehmigung beantragen | to apply for approval |

4 Beratungspraxis – Consultation

| Rx-bezogene Begriffe | Rx-related terms |
|---|---|
| Erstattung | reimbursement |
| etw. begründen | to justify sth. |
| etw. scannen | to scan sth. |
| etw. wird übernommen/abgedeckt (z. B. von der Krankenkasse) | to be covered by (e. g. the health insurance) |
| Festbeträge für Hilfsmittel | reference prices for therapeutic appliances |
| Firmenname | brand name |
| Generikum | generic drug |
| Großhändler | wholesale supplier |
| gültiges Rezept | valid prescription |
| Gültigkeit | validity |
| Import | import |
| importiert | to be imported |
| Kostenerstattung beantragen | to request a cost reimbursement |
| Krankenversicherung | health insurance |
| limitiert sein | to be limited |
| Mehrkosten | additional cost/charges/surcharges |
| Menge/Dosiseinheiten | total quantity/dosage units |
| Original | original |
| Packungsdesign | package design |
| Parallel-Import | parallel import |
| Rabattvertrag | discount agreement |
| Rechnung | invoice |
| Rezeptanforderungen | prescription requirements |
| Rezeptgebühr | prescription charge |
| Siegel | seal |
| ungültiges Rezept | invalid prescription |
| Unverträglichkeit | incompatibility |
| verfallen | to expire |
| Verfallsdatum | expiration date |
| Zahlung | payment |
| Zertifikat | certificate |

## II Die Beratung – The consultation

| Hinweise/Fragen | hints/questions |
|---|---|
| Haben Sie eine Kundenkarte? | Do you have a customer card? In German this refers to one's data being saved in the Pharmacy software system. |
| Für wen ist das Arzneimittel? | For whom is this/the medication? |
| Sind Sie mit der Anwendung des Arzneimittels vertraut? | Are you familiar with the usage of your medication? |
| Wissen Sie, wie Sie das Arzneimittel einnehmen sollen? | Do you know how to take the medication? |
| Wissen Sie, wofür dieses Arzneimittel ist? | Do you know what the medication is for? |
| Welche Erfahrungen haben Sie mit diesem Arzneimittel? | What experiences have you made with this medicine? |
| Wofür wenden Sie das Arzneimittel an? | What are you using XY for? |
| Gibt es noch etwas, was Sie über ihr neues Arzneimittel wissen möchten? | Is there anything else you would like to know about your new medicine? |
| Gibt es noch etwas, was Sie nochmal durchgehen möchten? | Is there anything you would like me to go over again? |
| Haben Sie das Gefühl, dass XY wirkt/Ihnen hilft? | Do you feel XY is working? |
| Wie kommen Sie mit XY zurecht? | How are you getting on with XY? |
| Können Sie mir sagen, warum XY Ihnen verschrieben wurde? | Can you tell me why XY has been prescribed for you? |
| Anhand Ihres Rezeptes sehe ich, dass Ihnen XY verschrieben wurde. | I see from your prescription you have been prescribed XY. |
| Ich würde Ihnen gerne einige Fragen stellen, um sicherzugehen, dass Sie XY richtig anwenden. Ist das für Sie ok? | I would like to ask you a few questions to make sure you know how to take your medication the right way. Is that ok with you? |
| Bitte halten Sie sich an die Anweisung. Dann wird alles gut. | Please stick to the instructions. You will be fine then. |
| Ich kann das nicht später als 28 Tage nach dem Ausstellungsdatum abgeben. | I cannot dispense this later than 28 days after the date of issue. |
| Ich muss mit Ihrem Arzt sprechen. | I have to talk to your medical doctor (NZ)/general practitioner (UK)/physician (U.S.A.). |
| Ihre Krankenkasse schreibt die Bedingungen vor. | Your health insurance will stipulate the terms. |
| Ihre Krankenkasse übernimmt/bezahlt nur diese Arzneimittelfirma/Arzneimittelfirmen. | Your health insurance covers only this brand/these medicinal brands. |
| Der Arzt hat Ihnen XY verschrieben. | The doctor has prescribed XY for you. |
| Der Arzt muss die Änderung gegenzeichnen. | The doctor has to sign the amendment. |

| Hinweise/Fragen | hints/questions |
|---|---|
| Die Abgabe von XY wird erstattet (durch die Krankenkasse). | The dispensing of XY will be reimbursed (by the health Insurance). |
| Das (XY) enthält exakt den gleichen Wirkstoff und die gleiche Stärke und Stückzahl. | This (XY) contains the exact same active ingredient/substance and the same dose/strength and quantity. |

### Beispiel – example

Y: *The doctor has prescribed Bisoprolol for you. Are you familiar with its usage?*
*(If the patient would like to know why the name on the medicine pack differs from the given name on the prescription again...)*
Y: *This medicine contains the exact substance Bisoprolol with the same strength and quantity. This is only a different brand. Your health insurance has a discount agreement with this brand and requests me to dispense it to you.*

S: Der Arzt hat Ihnen Bisoprolol verschrieben. Sind Sie mit der Anwendung vertraut?
(Wenn der Patient wissen will, warum der Name auf der Verpackung mal wieder anders heißt als auf dem Rezept...)
S: Dieses Medikament enthält den gleichen Wirkstoff Bisoprolol in der gleichen Stärke und Menge. Das ist nur eine andere Firma. Ihre Krankenkasse führt mit dieser Firma einen Rabattvertrag und schreibt vor, es abzugeben.

# 5 Beratungsthemen – Counseling topics

## 5.1 Erkältung – Common cold

In diesen Tabellen sind Begriffe und Formulierungen zur Therapie der Erkältung sowie den Symptomen Husten, Schnupfen und Schmerzen aufgelistet.

Within the tables below you will find expressions and phrases that are relevant for the treatment of the common cold as well as the symptoms cough, blocked nose and pain.

Hilfreiche Begriffe – Helpful terms

| Symptome | symptoms |
| --- | --- |
| Gliederschmerzen | body aches |
| Halsschmerzen | sore throat |
| Husten | cough |
| Kopfschmerzen | headache |
| leichtes Fieber | low-grade fever (more common in children) |
| Muskelschmerzen | myalgias |
| Nasenausfluss | runny nose/rhinorrhea |
| Nasenschleimhautentzündung | rhinitis |
| Niesen | sneezing |
| Postnasal-Drip-Syndrom (Nasensekretüberproduktion) | postnasal drip |
| Unwohlsein | mailaise |
| verstopfte Nase | nasal congestion/blocked or stuffy nose |

| Charakteristika | characteristics |
|---|---|
| Infekt der oberen Atemwege | upper respiratory tract infection (URI) |
| selbstlimitierend | self-limiting |
| virale/bakterielle Infektionen | viral/bacterial infections |

> **Beispiel – example**
>
> *The common cold is self-limiting in nature.*
> Die Erkältung ist in ihrer Natur selbst-limitierend.

## 5.1.1 Husten – Cough

In den untenstehenden Tabellen sind Begriffe und Formulierungen zur Therapie des Hustens aufgelistet. Relevante Fragen sind chronologisch, wie man Sie auch im Beratungsgespräch stellen würde, aufgeführt.

Within the tables below you will find expressions and phrases that are relevant for the cough treatment. Questions that you would ask during a consultation are being listed chronologically.

Hilfreiche Begriffe – Helpful terms

| Hustenarten | types of cough |
|---|---|
| akuter Husten* (< 3 Wochen) | acute cough* (< 3 weeks) |
| subakuter Husten (3–8 Wochen) | subacute cough (3–8 weeks) |
| chronischer Husten (> 8 Wochen) | chronic cough (> 8 weeks) |
| produktiver Husten | wet/moist cough |
| nicht-produktiver Husten/(trockener) Reizhusten | dry cough |

*Husten kann unterschiedlich eingeteilt werden (z. B. nach Dauer oder Ursache). Die Einteilung nach Sekretion (produktiv vs. nicht-produktiv) erfolgt bei erwachsenen Patienten aufgrund der Verwechslungsgefahr eigentlich nicht mehr. Da dies allerdings noch häufig in der Apotheke vorkommt, wurde es an dieser Stelle erwähnt.[9]
Cough can be classified into different types (e. g. based on duration or cause). The classification based on secretion (productive vs. non-productive) is no longer carried out for adult patients due to the risk of misinterpretation. Since it is however still commonly used in Pharmacies, it is listed as well.

---

9 Arbeitsgemeinschaft der Wissenschaftlichen Medizinischen Fachgesellschaften (AWMF) (Hg.) (2019): S2k-Leitlinie Diagnostik und Therapie von erwachsenen Patienten mit Husten. Online verfügbar unter https://register.awmf.org/de/leitlinien/detail/020-003, zuletzt aktualisiert am 01.01.2019, zuletzt geprüft am 18.01.2023

II Die Beratung – The consultation

| Ursachen/Auslöser (Auswahl) | causes/triggers (selection) |
|---|---|
| Arzneimittel-Einnahme (z. B. ACE-Hemmer, Gliptine) | drug-administration/intake (e. g. ACE-inhibitors, gliptins) |
| zugrundeliegende Erkrankung(en) (z. B. Asthma, chronisch obstruktive Lungenerkrankung (COPD), gastroösophageale Refluxkrankheit (GERD)) | underlying disease(s) (e. g. asthma, chronic obstructive pulmonary disease (COPD), gastroesophageal reflux disease (GERD)) |
| Hustenreiz | urge to cough/tickling in the throat |
| Irritation der Atemwege | irritation of the airways |
| Hustenreflex | cough reflex |
| **bakterielle/virale Infektion(en)** | **bacterial/viral infection(s)** |
| Bakterium | bacterium |
| Virus | virus |

| Art der Verbreitung des Erregers | mode of transmission of the pathogen |
|---|---|
| Tröpfcheninfektion | droplet infection |
| Schmierinfektion | smear infection |
| Aerosol(e)/über die Luft | aerosol(s)/via air |
| direkter/enger Kontakt | direct/close contact |

| Grenzen der Selbstmedikation (Auswahl) | when to refer to a medical doctor |
|---|---|
| Atemnot | shortness of breath/dyspnoea/difficulty in breathing |
| Aufenthalt in Tuberkulose-Gebieten/Kontakt zu einer infizierten Person | stay in tuberculosis areas/contact with infected people |
| Haben Sie sich in der letzten Zeit in einem Tuberkulose-Gebiet aufgehalten und/oder Kontakt zu potenziell Infizierten gehabt? | Have you recently stayed in a tuberculosis area and/or have had contact to potentially infected people? |
| blutiger Husten | bloody cough |
| Fieber | fever |
| Heiserkeit | hoarseness/croakiness |
| Husten, der länger als 8 Wochen andauert | cough present for more than 8 weeks |
| ungewöhnliche Hustengeräusche | unusual cough sounds |
| einen Verdacht haben, dass der Husten durch XY ausgelöst werden könnte | to have a suspicion that the cough is caused by XY |
| (stechender) Schmerz im Brustbereich/Thoraxschmerz | (sharp/stabbing) pain in the chest area/chest pain |

## Therapie des Hustens – Cough treatment

| Wirkstoffklassen | drug-classes |
|---|---|
| Antitussivum/Antitussiva/hustendämpfende/antitussive Hustenstiller (z. B. Dextrometorphan) | antitussives/cough suppressant(s) (e. g. Dextromethorphan) |
| Demulzenz/Demulzentien/reizlindernde Arzneimittel (z. B. Honig) | demulcent(s) (e. g. honey) |
| Expektoranz/Expektorantien/auswurffördernde/expektorationsfördernde Hustenmittel/»Hustenlöser« | expectorant(s) |
| Mukolytikum/Mukolytika (z. B. Ambroxol) | mucolytic(s) (e. g. Ambroxol) |
| • reduzieren die Schleimviskosität | • reduce mucus viscosity |
| Sekretolytikum/Sekretolytika (z. B. Ätherische-Öl-Drogen (z. B. Eukalyptus-Öl), z. B. saponinhaltige Drogen (z. B. Efeublätter)) | secretolytic(s) (e. g. essential oil/ethereal oil drugs (e. g. eucalyptus oil), e.g. saponine-drugs (e.g. ivy leaf extract)) |
| • erhöhen das Sekretvolumen/setzen die Oberflächenspannung des Schleims herab | • increase the secretion volume/decrease the surface tension of the mucus |
| Sekretomotorikum/Sekretomotorika (z. B. Thymiankraut) | secretomotoric agent(s) (e. g. thyme leaves) |
| • erleichtern den Bronchialschleimabtransport | • improve mucus evacuation |
| synthetische/chemische Substanzen | synthetic substances/chemical substances |
| pflanzliche Substanzen/Phytotherapeutika | herbal substances/phytotherapeutics |
| Hustenmittel | cough remedy |
| **Eigenschaften der/des Wirkstoffs/Wirkstoffe** | **properties of the active ingredient(s)** |
| antibakteriell | antibacterial |
| antientzündlich/anti-inflammatorisch | antiphlogistic/anti-inflammatory |
| antiviral | antiviral |
| entkrampfender Effekt | antispasmodic effect |
| lindernde/beruhigende Wirkung | soothing effect |
| das Abhusten erleichtern | to ease/facilitate expectoration |
| die Atemwege frei machen | to free the airways |
| (den) Schleim lösen | to loosen the mucus/phlegm; to dissolve slime |

II Die Beratung – The consultation

| Eigenschaften der/des Wirkstoffs/Wirkstoffe | properties of the active ingredient(s) |
|---|---|
| den Hustenreiz/Stimulus unterdrücken | to suppress the cough stimuli |
| Schleimverflüssigung | liquefaction of mucus |
| Sekretion von XY (z. B. Schleim) | secretion of XY (e. g. mucus) |
| die Schleimsekretion anregen | to increase mucus secretion |
| Verflüssigen von Schleim | liquefying of sputum/phlegm |
| die bronchiale Schleimsekretion stimulieren | to stimulate bronchial mucus secretion |

| allgemeine Sätze/Fragen zur Therapie des Hustens | general phrases/questions related to cough therapy |
|---|---|
| Wie äußert sich der Husten bei Ihnen? | How does the cough manifest itself? |
| Seit wann haben Sie diesen Husten? | Since when are you experiencing this cough? |
| Wann hat der Husten angefangen? | When did the cough start? |
| Hat der Husten plötzlich oder schleichend eingesetzt? | Was the onset of the cough sudden or gradual? |
| Ist der Husten trocken oder produktiv? | Is the cough dry or productive? |
| Welche Farbe hat der Schleim? | What colour is the phlegm? |
| Wann haben Sie den Husten hauptsächlich? (nachts/tagsüber) | When does the cough mainly occur? (during the day/night?) |
| Haben Sie auch andere Symptome? | Are you experiencing other symptoms as well? |
| Können Sie andere Ursachen für Ihren Husten ausschließen? (Zum Beispiel eine allergische Rhinitis) | Can you exclude other causes of your cough? (e. g. an allergic rhinitis) |
| Es ist wichtig die Ursache für Ihren Husten zu behandeln. | It is important to treat the underlying cause of your cough. |
| Sodbrennen, Allergien oder bestimmte Medikamente, wie z. B. Blutdruckmedikamente, können einen Husten auslösen. | Acid reflux, allergies or certain medications such as blood pressure drugs for instance may also cause a cough. |
| Es ist wichtig, die Ursache für Ihren Husten zu behandeln. | It is important to treat the underlying cause of your cough. |
| Wie haben Sie den Husten bisher behandelt? | How did you treat the cough so far? |

## 5 Beratungsthemen – Counseling topics

| Therapieempfehlungen | treatment recommendations |
|---|---|
| Anhand der Beschreibung Ihrer Symptome empfehle ich Ihnen, XY einzunehmen. | Based on the description of your symptoms, I recommend taking XY. |
| XY ist ein Mukolytikum/Schleimlöser, der das Abhusten erleichtert. | XY is a mucolytic, that will loosen the phlegm and ease expectoration. |
| Den Hustenlöser nimmt man 3-mal täglich nach einer Mahlzeit ein. | One takes the expectorant 3 times daily after a meal. |
| Die Hustentropfen bitte in einem Glas Wasser auflösen und vor Einnahme vermischen. | Please dissolve the cough drops in a glass of water and shake it before the intake. |
| Diese Kapseln enthalten einen hochkonzentrierten Wirkstoff mit einer speziellen Formulierung. Die Kapseln geben über den Tag verteilt einen Wirkstoff frei, der Ihren Husten löst. Nehmen Sie bitte nur eine Kapsel morgens nach dem Frühstück ein. | These capsules contain a highly concentrated active substance in a special formulation. These capsules release the active ingredient that will help relieve your cough throughout the day. Please take only one capsule after breakfast. |
| Die Kapseln bitte spätestens bis XY Uhr einnehmen, da Sie sonst in der Nacht den Schleim abhusten müssen. | Please take the capsules until XY p.m., you will have to cough up the mucus at night otherwise. |
| Wenn Sie den Hustenstiller und den Hustenlöser gleichzeitig einnehmen, kann es zu einem Sekretstau kommen. | If you take the cough suppressant and the expectorant simultaneously/at the same time, you can cause a secretion congestion. |
| Bitte nehmen Sie den Hustenstiller nur zur Nacht ein. | Please take the cough suppressant at night time only. |
| Vor der Einnahme sollte man den Hustensaft schütteln, damit sich alle Stoffe gleich verteilen. | Shake the linctus before the intake, because all the substances need to be spread equally. |
| In diesen Hustentropfen ist ein ethanolischer Pflanzenextrakt enthalten. Die Tropfen enthalten somit Alkohol. | These cough drops contain an ethanolic plant extract and therefore alcohol. |
| Wenn Sie merken, dass der Husten in 1 bis 2 Wochen nicht besser wird, sollten Sie einen Arzt aufsuchen oder sich gerne nochmal an uns wenden. | If the cough does not stop within the next 2 weeks, please visit a doctor or feel free to get in touch with us again. |

| nicht medikamentöse Zusatzmaßnahmen | non-medical measures |
|---|---|
| (Dampf-)Inhalation(en) | (steam) inhalation(s) |
| (Husten-)Bonbons lutschen | to suck on candy/cough drops |
| Badezusatz mit ätherischem Öl/ein Bad nehmen | bath additive with ethereal oils/to take a bath |
| Einreibung (mit ätherischem Öl) | rub/embrocation (with aetherical oils) |

## II Die Beratung – The consultation

| nicht medikamentöse Zusatzmaßnahmen | non-medical measures |
|---|---|
| das Immunsystem stärken | to strengthen/boost your immune system |
| sich ausruhen/körperliche Anstrengung vermeiden | to rest/to relax/to avoid physical strain/to avoid physical exertion |
| Tee(-aufguss) | tea (infusion) |
| die Nase durchspülen | to rinse your nose |
| (mit z. B. Salzwasser) gurgeln | to gargle (with e. g. saltwater) |

| Behandlung anderer oder assoziierter Symptome/Anzeichen | treatment of other or associated symptoms/signs |
|---|---|
| Erkältung | cold/common cold |
| Entzündung | inflammation |
| eitriges/blutiges/visköses Sekret | purulent/bloody/viscous sputum |
| Infektion | infection |
| Schmerz(en)/Gliederschmerzen | pain/limb pain/aching limbs |
| Schnupfen | blocked/stuffy nose/head cold |
| Sputum/Auswurf/abgehustetes schleimiges Sekret | sputum/phlegm |
| Schleim | mucus/phlegm/slime |
| Halskratzen | sore throat |
| bakterielle Superinfektion | bacterial superinfection |

| allgemeine Begriffe/Beispielsätze | general terms |
|---|---|
| akute/allgemeine Bronchitis | acute bronchitis/chest cold |
| Atemweg(e) | airway(s)/respiratory tract/air passage |
| Dosierkappe | dosage cap/dosing cap |
| Dosierpipette/Dosierspritze | dosing pipette/dosing syringe |
| Erkältungsmittel | cold remedy |
| hartnäckig | persistent |
| Husten in der Nacht/nachts wachhalten | night-time cough/to keep you up at night |
| Hustenrezeptoren | cough receptors |
| Hustensaft | linctus |
| Hustentropfen | cough drops |

## 5 Beratungsthemen – Counseling topics

| allgemeine Begriffe/Beispielsätze | general terms |
|---|---|
| Keuchhusten | whooping cough |
| Linderung von | relief of |
| Lunge | lungs |
| Lungenerkrankung | airway disease |
| Medikamenten-induzierter Husten | medication induced cough |
| obere Atemwege | upper airways |
| Sekretstau | congestion |
| untere Atemwege | lower airways |

**Beispiel – example**

Y: *You said you have a cough. How does it manifest itself?*
C: *I have had this dry cough for approximately 2 days. It started off with a scratchy throat.*
Y: *Are you experiencing any other symptoms?*

S: Sie sagen Sie haben Husten, wie äußert sich der Husten bei Ihnen?
K: Ich habe seit ca. 2 Tagen diesen trockenen Reizhusten. Es fing mit einem Halskratzen an.
S: Haben Sie noch andere Symptome?

### 5.1.2 Schnupfen – Stuffy/blocked nose

In diesem Kapitel finden Sie Begriffe rund um das Thema Schnupfen. Da man Kunden mit Nasenspray-Abhängigkeit auch häufig im Apothekenalltag begegnet, wurden auch hierzu Begriffe und Formulierungen aufgelistet.

In this chapter, you will find cold-related expressions and phrases. Since one encounters nasal-spray dependent clients frequently in community pharmacies, related expressions and phrases were included as well.

Hilfreiche Begriffe – Helpful terms

| Ort der Beschwerden | location of discomforts |
|---|---|
| angeschwollenener Nasengang | swollen nasal passage |
| Flimmerepithel | ciliated epithelium |
| Nasenloch | nostril |
| Nasennebenhöhle | paranasal sinus |

| Ort der Beschwerden | location of discomforts |
| --- | --- |
| Nasenschleimhaut | mucous membrane |
| Schleimhautepithel | mucous membrane epithelium |
| Schläfe | temple |

| Beschwerden | discomfort |
| --- | --- |
| allergischer (allergiebedingter) Schnupfen | allergic rhinitis |
| dauerhaft angeschwollene Nasenschleimhaut | permanently swollen mucous membrane |
| Nasennebenhöhlenentzündung/Sinusitis | (nasal) sinusitis |
| Nasenschleimhautentzündung | rhinitis |
| Niesen | to sneeze/sneezing |
| Niesreiz | urge to sneeze |
| trockene Nasenschleimhaut | dry mucous membrane |
| verstopfte Nase | stuffy nose/blocked nose |
| wunde Nase | sore nose |
| Druckgefühl | feeling of pressure |
| Druckkopfschmerz | sinus headache |

| Therapie | therapy |
| --- | --- |
| Abschwellen der Nasenschleimhaut | decongestion of the mucous membrane |
| abschwellendes Nasenspray | decongestant nasal spray |
| α-Sympathomimetika (*Xylometazolin*) | α-adrenergic agonists (*Xylometazoline*) |
| Sekretlösung | liquefaction of the secretion |
| Dieses Nasenspray enthält einen Wirkstoff, der Ihre Schleimhaut abschwellen lässt. | This nasal spray contains a substance that decongests your mucous membrane. |
| Dieses Nasenspray können Sie bis zu 3-mal täglich im Abstand von XY Stunden anwenden. | You can use this nasal spray up to 3 times daily at intervals of XY hours. |
| Bitte über Kreuz in jedes Nasenloch applizieren. | Please apply the nasal spray crosswise into each nostril. |
| Wenn Sie Nasensprays nicht häufig anwenden, können Sie auch die Dosierung für Kinder verwenden. Bei Bedarf können Sie die Dosierung auf je 2 Sprühstöße erhöhen. | If you do not use nasal sprays often, you can apply the dosage that is recommended for children. In case of need you can increase the dosage to up to 2 sprays per nostril. |

## 5 Beratungsthemen – Counseling topics

| Therapie | therapy |
|---|---|
| Dieses Nasenspray können Sie bis zu 5 Tage lang anwenden. | You can use this nasal spray up to 5 days. |
| Das im Nasenspray enthaltende Konservierungsmittel kann die Schleimhaut Ihrer Nase schädigen. | The nasal spray contains a preservative that may damage your mucous membrane. |
| Ich suche Ihnen gerne ein Konservierungsmittel-freies Nasenspray heraus. | I am happy to select a preservative-free nasal spray for you. |
| Für Kinder ≤ 2 Jahren stehen Nasentropfen zur Verfügung. | For children aged ≤ 2 there are nasal drops available. |
| In Ihrem Falle empfehle ich ein Nasenspray, das zusätzlich eine pflegende Komponente enthält (z. B. *Dexpanthenol*). | In your case I recommend taking a nasal spray that contains an additional soothing component (e. g. *Dexpanthenol*). |
| Zur Lösung des Schleimes in den Nasennebenhöhlen können Sie zudem noch XY einnehmen. | In order to liquefy the mucous in your sinuses you can take XY as well. |
| Bitte 1 Kapsel/Tablette ca. eine halbe Stunde vor der Mahlzeit mit einem Glas Wasser einnehmen. | Please take 1 capsule/tablet with a glass of water approximately half an hour before your meal. |

| Nasenspray-Abhängigkeit | nasal spray addiction/nasal spray dependency |
|---|---|
| Rebound-Effekt | rebound-effect |
| Wenn Sie das Nasenspray zu lange anwenden, kommt es zum reflektorischen Anschwellen Ihrer Nasenschleimhaut. Das bedeutet, dass die Nase automatisch verstopft ist. | If you use the nasal spray for too long, a reflectory swelling of the mucous membrane will occur. This means that your nose will automatically be blocked. |
| Zur Entwöhnung können Sie zunächst die Dosis reduzieren. Anstatt des 0,1 %igen können Sie ein 0,05 %iges abschwellendes Nasenspray anwenden. Anschließend können Sie auf ein Meerwasser-haltiges Nasenspray umsteigen. | For a withdrawal you can decrease the dosage by taking a 0,05 % instead of a 0,1 % concentrated decongesting nasal spray. Afterwards you can switch to a sea water-based nasal spray. |
| Gewebe schädigen/zerstören | to damage/destroy tissue |

| nicht medikamentöse Maßnahmen | non-pharmacologic treatment |
|---|---|
| Meerwasserspray | sea water nasal spray |
| osmotischer Effekt | osmotic effect |
| Befeuchtung der Nasenschleimhaut | moistening of the mucous membrane |
| 0,9 % (isotone) Kochsalzlösung/Natriumchlorid-Lösung/NaCl-Lösung | 0,9 % (isotonic) saline (solution)/sodium chloride solution/NaCl-solution |

II Die Beratung – The consultation

| nicht medikamentöse Maßnahmen | non-pharmacologic treatment |
|---|---|
| Die Nase durchspülen | to rinse your sinus/nose |
| hypertone Lösung | hypertonic solution |
| Nasendusche | sinus rinse/sinus flush |
| Nasenpflege | nasal care |
| Rauchkarenz/Rauchen vermeiden | smoking abstinence/to avoid smoking |
| Raumluft befeuchten | to humidify the air |

**Beispiel – example**

C: *Hello, I would like to purchase a nasal spray, because I have a cold and my nose is blocked. At night I have trouble breathing and would like to get a good night's sleep.*
Y: *How long have you had the stuffy nose?*
C: *For 2 days. I fortunately do not have a stuffy nose very often. I also have no allergies. Your colleague recommended a decongestant, preservative-free nasal spray last time, which really helped.*

K: Guten Tag, ich würde gerne ein Nasenspray kaufen, da meine Nase zu ist, weil ich Schnupfen habe. Ich bekomme besonders nachts schlecht Luft und möchte endlich wieder durchschlafen.
S: Seit wann haben Sie den Schnupfen?
K: Seit 2 Tagen. Schnupfen habe ich zum Glück nicht oft. Ich habe auch keine Allergien. Letztes Mal hatte mir ihr Kollege ein abschwellendes, konservierungsmittelfreies Nasenspray empfohlen. Das hat sehr gut geholfen.

## 5.1.3 (Kopf-)Schmerzen – Headache/pain

In den Tabellen sind Begriffe und Formulierungen zum Thema aufgeführt. Der Hauptfokus liegt auf der Behandlung von Kopfschmerzen und Migräne in der Selbstmedikation.

Within the tables you will find terms and phrases that are associated with pain. The main focus lies on the self-medication treatment of headaches and migraines.

## Hilfreiche Begriffe – Helpful terms

| Schmerzarten/Ort des Schmerzes (Auswahl) | types of pain/site of pain (selection) |
|---|---|
| Schmerzen | pain |
| Abdominalschmerzen/Unterleibsschmerzen/Bauchschmerzen | abdominal pain |
| Beckenschmerzen | pelvic pain |
| Brustschmerzen | chest pain |
| Gliederschmerzen | limb pain/body aches |
| Halsschmerzen | sore throat |
| Herzschmerzen | heartaches |
| Kopfschmerzen | headache |
| Clusterkopfschmerz | cluster headache |
| Migräne(-kopfschmerz) (mit Aura) | migraine (with aura) |
| Spannungskopfschmerzen | tension-type headache |
| Menstruationsbeschwerden/Periodenschmerzen | menstrual pains/period pains |
| Muskelschmerzen/Myalgie | muscle pains/muscle soreness/myalgia |
| Ohrenschmerzen | earache/otalgia |
| Rückenschmerzen | back pain |
| Schulterschmerzen | shoulder pain |
| Nackenschmerzen | neck pain |
| Tumorschmerzen | tumor pain |
| Zahnschmerzen | toothache |

| Art des Schmerzes | nature of pain |
|---|---|
| ausstrahlen | to radiate |
| Dumpf | dull |
| ganzseitig/halbseitig (in Bezug auf Kopfschmerzen) | bilateral/unilateral |
| plötzlich | sudden |
| pochend | throbbing |
| pulsierend | pulsating |
| stechend | stabbing/stinging |

| Dauer | duration |
|---|---|
| akut | acute |
| chronisch | chronic |
| permanent | permanent |
| vorrübergehend | temporary |

| Begleitsymptome | associated symptoms |
|---|---|
| Appetitlosigkeit | loss of appetite |
| Lichtempfindlichkeit | photophobia/being sensitive to light |
| Nackensteifigkeit | neck stiffness |
| Schwindel | vertigo/dizziness |
| Übelkeit | nausea |
| Erbrechen | vomit |

## Therapie (Auswahl) – Therapy

Analgetika – Analgetics

| nicht saure non-opioid Analgetika | non-acidic non-opioid analgetics |
|---|---|
| *Paracetamol (Paracetamol-ratiopharm®)* | *Paracetamol/Acetaminophen (Tylenol®)* |
| *Metamizol* | *Metamizole/Dipyrone* |
| **nichtsteroidale Antiphlogistika (NSAID)** | **non-steroidal anti-inflammatory drugs (NSAIDs)** |
| selektive Cyclooxygenase (COX)-2-Hemmer (*Celecoxib*) | selective cyclooxygenase (COX)-2-inhibitors (*Cyclocoxib*) |
| **unselektive Cyclooxygenase (COX)-Hemmer** | **non-selective cyclooxygenase-inhibitors** |
| *Acetylsalicylsäure* | *Acetylsalicylic acid* |
| *Diclofenac* | *Diclofenac* |
| *Ibuprofen* | *Ibuprofen* |
| *Indometacin* | *Indomethacin* |
| *Naproxen* | *Naproxen* |

## 5 Beratungsthemen – Counseling topics

## Sonstige Wirkstoffe – Other agents

| | |
|---|---|
| »Kombinationsmittel« *(Ibuprofen + Koffein)* | combined remedies *(Ibuprofen + Coffein)* |
| Triptane/Serotonin-5HT1B/1D-Agonisten *(Naratriptan)* | triptans/serotonin-5HT1B/1D agonists *(Naratriptan)* |
| *pflanzliche Schmerzmittel* | *plant-based pain killers* |
| Arnika | Arnica |
| Beinwell | Comfrey |
| Menthol | Menthol |
| Teufelskralle | Devil's claw |

| Wirkstoffeigenschaften | properties of the active substance(s) |
|---|---|
| antiphlogistisch/entzündungshemmend | antiphlogistic/anti-inflammatory |
| fiebersenkend | antipyretic |
| schmerzstillend | analgesic/pain-relieving |

## Beratung bei Kopfschmerzen – Headache counseling

| Hinweise und Fragen | additional hints and questions |
|---|---|
| Wie fühlen sich Ihre Kopfschmerzen an? | How does your headache feel? |
| Seit wann haben Sie diese Kopfschmerzen? | When did you begin experiencing these headaches? |
| Haben Sie bereits etwas zur Schmerzstillung eingenommen? | Have you taken something yet to relieve the pain? |
| Werden die Kopfschmerzen bei Bewegung schlimmer? | Do the headaches get worse when you exercise? |
| Haben Sie Vorerkrankungen? | Do you have any pre-existing conditions/underlying health conditions? |
| Können Sie eine Schwangerschaft zurzeit ausschließen?/Sie sollten das Arzneimittel nicht einnehmen, wenn Sie schwanger sind. Im Falle einer Schwangerschaft.../(Ich muss Sie leider fragen ...) | Can you currently exclude a pregnancy?/You should not take this medicine in case you are pregnant. In case of a pregnancy.../(I am afraid I have to ask ...) |
| Asthma oder »Magenprobleme« liegen nicht vor? | Asthma or gastric problems are not present? |
| Ich empfehle Ihnen XY, um die Schmerzen zu mildern. | I recommend you to take XY to ease the pain. |

105

II Die Beratung – The consultation

| Hinweise und Fragen | additional hints and questions |
|---|---|
| Sie können bis zu 3 Tabletten in 24 Stunden im Abstand von 8 Stunden einnehmen. | You can take up to 3 tablets within 24 hours. Take one tablet every 8 hours. |
| Sollte der Schmerz nicht nachlassen, können Sie eine weitere Tablette einnehmen. | If the pain does not alleviate, you can take another tablet. |
| Bitte nehmen Sie die Tabletten nicht länger als XY (z. B. 3 aufeinander folgende ) Tage ein und insgesamt nicht mehr als 10 Tage im Monat. | Please do not take the tablets for more than XY (e. g. 3 consecutive) days and more than 10 days per month in total. |
| Die Dosierung richtet sich nach dem Körpergewicht. | The dosage depends on your body weight. |
| Sie können Ihrem Kind eine Tablette/ein Zäpfchen innerhalb von 8 Stunden geben. | You can give your child a tablet/suppository within 8 hours. |
| Sie sollten danach einen Arzt aufsuchen, um die Ursache Ihres Schmerzes herauszufinden. | You should see a doctor to find out about the cause of your pain afterwards. |
| Sollten Sie nicht zufriedenstellend auf das Schmerzmittel ansprechen, muss ich Sie an einen Arzt verweisen. | If you do not respond satisfactorily to the pain killer, I have to refer you to a medical doctor. |
| Bei Migräne: Wurde die Migräne durch einen Arzt diagnostiziert? | When dealing with migraine: Has the migraine been diagnosed by a doctor? |
| Bei Triptanen: Wenn Sie auf die erste Dosis nicht ansprechen, sollten Sie auf keinen Fall eine weitere Dosis einnehmen. | When taking triptans: If you do not respond to the first dosage, you should not take another one. |
| Nehmen Sie nicht mehr als 2 Tabletten innerhalb von 24 Stunden zur Behandlung des gleichen Anfalls ein. | Do not exceed taking more than 2 tablets within 24 hours during the same attack. |
| Ich sehe anhand Ihrer Medikation, dass Sie ein Antikoagulanz/Medikament »zur Blutverdünnung« einnehmen. Wenn Sie zusätzlich dieses Schmerzmittel einnehmen, kann sich dieser Effekt verstärken. | Based on your medication I see that you are taking an anticoagulant/«blood thinning medication«. If you additionally take this pain killer, this effect may be amplified. |
| Während der Stillzeit sollte man XY nicht einnehmen, da es in die Muttermilch übergehen kann. | XY should not be taken during the breastfeeding period as it can be excreted into the breast milk. |
| Ibuprofen wird hauptsächlich über die Niere ausgeschieden. | Ibuprofen is mainly excreted via the kidneys. |
| Paracetamol wird hauptsächlich über die Leber verstoffwechselt. | Paracetamol is mainly metabolised via the liver. |
| Bei Nierenfunktionsstörungen würde ich Ihnen dringend raten, stattdessen Paracetamol einzunehmen. | In case of renal dysfunction(s) I would strongly recommend you take Paracetamol instead. |

## 5 Beratungsthemen – Counseling topics

| Hinweise und Fragen | additional hints and questions |
|---|---|
| Ibuprofen könnte einen Asthma-Anfall auslösen. In ihrem Falle würde ich Ihnen eher Paracetamol empfehlen. | Ibuprofen could trigger an asthma-attack. In your case I would recommend rather taking Paracetamol. |
| Sie sollten ASS nicht einnehmen, wenn eine OP bevorsteht, da der Wirkstoff einen antikoagulierenden/»blutverdünnenden« Effekt hat, der i. d. R. 10 Tage anhält. | You should not take ASS in case you have an impending surgery as the active substance has an anticoagulant/«blood thinning« effect that lasts for approximately 10 days. |
| Wenn Sie Magenprobleme haben, sollten Sie die Tabletten nicht nüchtern einnehmen. | If you have gastric problems, you should not take the tablets on an empty stomach. |
| Ihrer Beschreibung zufolge haben Sie vermutlich eher Muskelverspannungen. Das Schmerzmittel könnte die Schmerzen maskieren aber nicht die Ursache bekämpfen. | According to your description, you seem to have strained a muscle. The pain killer may mask the pain but does not fight the cause. |
| Ich muss Sie leider an einen Arzt verweisen. Ihr/Ihre XY (z. B. Schwellung im Kopfbereich) sollte genauer untersucht werden. | I unfortunately have to refer you to a medical doctor. Your XY (e. g. swelling in the head area) needs to be further examined. |

| Zusatzmaßnahmen | additional measures |
|---|---|
| ausreichend Flüssigkeit | enough liquids |
| ausreichend Schlaf | enough sleep |
| Bewegung/regelmäßige Bewegung | exercise/constant exercise |
| Entspannungsübungen/Entspannungstechniken | relaxation techniques |
| regelmäßige Nahrungszufuhr | regular food intake |
| Vermeidung von Triggerfaktoren | avoidance of trigger factors |

| Allgemeine Begriffe | general terms |
|---|---|
| Alkohol-Einnahme | alcohol intake |
| Belastung/körperliche Anstrengung | physical exertion |
| Frequenz/Häufigkeit | frequency |
| Körperhaltung | posture |
| Magenblutungen | gastric bleeding/gastrostaxis |
| Magenreizung | gastric irritation |
| medikamenteninduzierter Kopfschmerz (MOH) | medication-induced headache (MIH)/medication overuse headache (MOH) |
| Medikamentenübergebrauch | medication overuse |

II Die Beratung – The consultation

| Allgemeine Begriffe | general terms |
|---|---|
| Schädel | skull |
| Schleimhautblutungen | mucosal bleeding |
| Schmerzempfinden | pain perception |
| Schmerzgedächtnis | pain memory |
| Schmerzlinderung | pain relief |
| schwere Lasten tragen/heben | to bear heavy burdens |
| sich im Laufe des Tages verbessern | to improve throughout the day |
| Stress | stress |
| Verletzung | injury (mild-moderate)/trauma (severe) |
| Verspannung/verspannt sein | tension |
| Zeitpunkt der Symptome | timing of symptoms |

**Beispiel – example**

*C: Hello. I am passing through and I have a headache since this morning. I need something that helps relieve the pain quickly.*
*Y: Hello. How does your headache feel?*

K: Hallo. Ich bin auf der Durchreise und habe heute Morgen Kopfschmerzen bekommen. Ich bräuchte Etwas, was den Schmerz schnell lindert.
S: Guten Tag. Wie fühlt sich der Kopfschmerz bei Ihnen an?

## 5.2 Impfungen und Reisekrankheiten – Vaccinations and travel-related diseases

In den Tabellen finden Sie hilfreiche Begriffe und Formulierungen rund um das Thema Impfungen und reisebedingte Krankheiten.

Within the tables below you will find expressions and phrases about vaccine and travel-related diseases.

## Erregerbezogene Begriffe – Pathogen-associated expressions

| | |
|---|---|
| Amöbe(n) | amoeba(s) |
| Bakterium/Bakterien (pl) | bacteria |
| der/das Virus | the virus |
| Pilz(e) | fungus |
| Wurm | worm |
| Zecke(n) | tick(s) |
| endemisch/heimisch (an einem Ort auftretend) | endemic |
| Expositionsrisiko/ Risiko sich XY auszusetzen/berufsbedingte Exposition | risk of exposure/exposure risk/risk of occupational exposure |
| reisebezogen | travel-related |
| Risikogebiet | risk area/region |
| Gesundheitspersonal/Laborpersonal | health/laboratory personnel |
| Vor Antritt der Reise sollten Sie sich (z. B.) im Tropeninstitut beraten lassen. | Prior to your travels/before your travels you can seek advice (e. g.) through the Institute of Tropical Medicine. |
| Sie können sich (z. B. auf der Website des auswärtigen Amtes) informieren. | You can inform yourself (e. g. on the Federal Foreign Office website) |
| Rat | advice |
| Institut für Tropenmedizin | Tropical Institute/Institute of Tropical Medicine |
| Weltgesundheitsorganisation (WHO) | World Health Organization (WHO) |
| **Immunantwort** | **immune response** |
| Antikörper | antibodies |
| seronegativ | seronegative |
| impfstoffassoziierter/s Schmerz/Fieber | vaccine associated pain/fever |
| Linderung der Beschwerden | alleviating discomfort |
| Symptome nach der Impfung | symptoms after vaccination |
| Immunstatus | Immune status |
| Immunogenität | immunogenicity |
| eine Immunantwort auslösen | to induce an immune response |
| Spritze | syringe |
| etw. (intramuskulär) injizieren | to inject sth (intramuscular) |

II Die Beratung – The consultation

| Immunantwort | immune response |
|---|---|
| nasale Applikation | nasal application |
| Prophylaxe | prophylaxis |
| langanhaltender/dauerhafter Impfschutz | long-lasting vaccination protection |
| Erreger/Keim/Virus/Bakterium | pathogen/germ/virus/bacteria |
| Inkubationszeit | incubation time/incubation period |
| Latenzzeit | latency (time/period) |
| Ansteckung | contagion/infection |
| ansteckend (sein) | (to be) contagious |

## Impfungen – Vaccinations

| Impfung(en) | vaccination/inoculation(s)/shot(s)/vaccine injection(s)/jab(s) |
|---|---|
| impfen/sich impfen lassen/gegen XY impfen | to vaccinate/to get/be vaccinated/ to vaccinate against/to inoculate |
| Schutz vor | protection against |
| einer Krankheit/Erkrankung XY vorbeugen | to prevent XY disease |
| Die/Das STIKO/CDC empfiehlt die Impfung ab den folgendem Alter [...] | The STIKO/CDC recommends shots at the following ages [...] |
| Grundimmunsierung | primary immunization (AE)/immunisation (BE) |
| Auffrischungsimpfung | booster vaccination/revaccination |
| Standardimpfung | standard vaccination |
| Impfpass | vaccination certificate/vaccination record/ vaccination card/immunisation record (BE)/ vaccine passport |
| Impfkalender | immunization schedule (AE)/immunisation schedule (BE) |
| Impfdokumentation | vaccination documentation |
| eine Impfung verabreichen | to administer a vaccine |
| Einmalimpfstoff | one-dose-vaccine/one-shot-vaccine |
| Impfschutz/Impfstoff-bedingter Schutz | vaccine-induced protection |
| aktive Immunisierung | active immunization (AE)/immunisation (BE) |
| passive Immunisierung | passive immunization (AE)/immunisation (BE) |

# 5 Beratungsthemen – Counseling topics

| | |
|---|---|
| (Impf-) Intervall/Abstand/Zeitspanne | (vaccination) interval |
| fehlende Impfdosis | missing vaccine dose |
| Bitte geben Sie den Impfstoff direkt an der Rezeption der Arztpraxis ab. | Please deliver your vaccine at the reception of the doctor's office immediately. |
| Kühltasche | cooler bag/cooling bag |
| Ich bestelle den Impfstoff gerne für Sie. | I am happy to order the vaccine for you. |
| Ich kann den Impfstoff leider nicht für Sie bestellen, da er zurzeit nicht verfügbar ist. | I unfortunately cannot order the vaccine for you, because it is out of stock/not available. |
| Diese Impfung können Sie direkt in der Arztpraxis/im Tropeninstitut bekommen. | You can get this vaccination at your local doctor's office/the Institute of Tropical Medicine. |
| auftauen (lassen) | to thaw |
| kühlpflichtig | obligatory refrigerated/requires cooling |
| Kühlkette | cooling chain |
| nicht schütteln | do not shake |
| Den Impfstoff bei XY °C lagern. | to store the vaccine at XY °C. |
| Impftermin | vaccination appointment |

## Impfung (gegen) – Vaccination (against)

| Standardimpfungen in Europa | standard vaccinations in Europe |
|---|---|
| Diphtherie | diphtheria |
| Haemophilus influenzae b (Hib) | haemophilus influenzae b (Hib) |
| Hepatitis B (HB) | hepatitis B (HB) |
| Humane Papillomaviren (HPV) | human papillomavirus (HPV) |
| Influenza, jährliche Grippeimpfung | influenza, »seasonal flu vaccine« |
| Masern | measles |
| Meningokokken (C, ACWY) | meningococcal C, ACWY (MenC, MenACWY) |
| Mumps, Röteln | mumps, rubella |
| Pertussis, »Keuchhusten« | pertussis, »whooping cough« |
| Pneumokokken | pneumococcus |
| Poliomyelitis (IPV) | poliomyelitis (IPV) |
| Rotavirus (RV) | rotavirus (RV) |
| Tetanus | tetanus |

II Die Beratung – The consultation

| Standardimpfungen in Europa | standard vaccinations in Europe |
|---|---|
| Varizellen (Symptom: Herpes Zoster/Gürtelrose/Windpocken) | varicella (symptom: shingles, chickenpox) |

| zusätzliche Impfungen (Auswahl) | additional vaccinations (selection) |
|---|---|
| Cholera | cholera |
| Frühsommer-Meningoenzephalitis (FSME) | tick-borne encephalitis (TBE) |
| Gelbfieber | yellow fever |
| Hepatitis A (HA) | hepatitis A (HA) |
| Japanische Enzephalitis | japanese encephalitis |
| Tollwut | rabies |
| Tuberkulose | tuberculosis |
| Typhoides Fieber/Typhus | typhoid fever |
| Typhus | typhus |

## Impftsoffarten – Types of vaccines

| Kombinationsimpfstoff(e) | combination vaccination(s) |
|---|---|
| (attenuierter/abgeschwächter) Lebendimpfstoff (z. B. Varizellen-Impfstoff) | live-attenuated vaccine (e. g. Varicella vaccine) |
| Totimpfstoff | inactivated/killed/dead vaccine |
| Ganzpartikelimpfstoff (z. B. Tollwut-Impfstoff) | inactivated vaccine/inactivated whole microorganism (e. g. Rabies vaccine) |
| Toxoidimpfstoff (z. B. Tetanus-Impfstoff) | toxoid vaccine (e. g. Tetanus vaccine) |
| Konjugatimpfstoff (z. B. Hib-Impfstoff) | conjugate vaccine (e. g. Hib-vaccine) |
| Polysaccharidimpfstoff (z. B. Pneumokokken-Impfstoff) | polysaccharide-based vaccine (e. g. Pneumococcus vaccine) |
| Subunit-Impfstoff (»Untereinheiten-Impfstoff«; Totimpfstoff mit Antigenen, oftmals auch »Protein-basiert«) (z. B. Hepatitis-B-Impfstoff) | subunit, recombinant, polysaccharide and conjugate vaccine/subunit vaccine/often »protein-based vaccine« (e. g. hepatitis B vaccine) |
| Adsorbatimpfstoff (z. B. Diphtherie-Tetanus-Impfstoff) | adsorbate vaccine (z. B. Diphtheria-Tetanus-vaccine) |
| genetische Impfstoffe | genetic vaccines |
| Vektorimpfstoff (z. B. Ebola-Impfstoff) | viral vector vaccine (e. g. ebola vaccine) |

| | |
|---|---|
| (m)RNA-Impfstoff (z. B. *COVID-19-Impfstoff*) | (messenger) RNA ((m)RNA) vaccine (e.g. *COVID-19 vaccine*) |
| DNA-Impfstoff (z. B. *COVID-19-Impfstoff*) | DNA-vaccine (e.g. *COVID-19 vaccine*) |

**Beispiel – example**

Y: *The doctor has prescribed a combination vaccine against Tetanus, Diphtheria and Pertussis for you. I assume this is your booster shot?*
C: *Yes, my last vaccination was approximately 10 years ago.*
Y: *Good. I am happy to order the vaccine for you. If you wish, we can also deliver it directly to your doctor's office so that you don't have to pick it up prior to your vaccination appointment and worry about refrigerating it.*
C: *That would be great.*

S: Der Arzt hat Ihnen einen Kombinationsimpfstoff gegen Tetanus, Diphtherie und Keuchhusten verschrieben. Ich nehme an, dass das Ihre Auffrischungsimpfung ist?
K: Ja, meine letzte Impfung ist ungefähr 10 Jahre her.
S: Gut. Ich kann Ihnen den Impfstoff gerne bestellen. Wenn Sie wünschen, können wir den Impfstoff auch direkt in die Arztpraxis liefern, damit Sie sich nicht um die Abholung vor Ihrem Impftermin und die kühle Lagerung kümmern müssen.

## 5.3 Notfallkontrazeption (»Pille danach«) – Emergency contraception (»morning-after pill«/ »emergency pill«)

In der untenstehenden Tabelle finden Sie Begriffe und Formulierungen, die für die Beratung und Abgabe von Notfallkontrazeptiva hilfreich sind. Die Chronologie der Begriffe und Formulierungen richtet sich nach dem Verlauf eines Beratungsgespräches.

In the table below you will find expressions and phrases that are of relevance for the consultation and dispense of emergency contraceptives. The order is based on the chronology of a typical conversation with a client.

II Die Beratung – The consultation

## Notfallkontrazeption – Emergency contraception

| | |
|---|---|
| persönliche Beratung | personal consultation |
| Ich muss Ihnen einige Fragen stellen, um zu prüfen, ob die Notfallkontrazeption für Sie geeignet ist. | I have to ask you a few questions in order to check whether the emergency pill is suitable for you. |
| Bitte folgen Sie mir (in den Beratungsraum/die Beratungsecke). | Please follow me (to our consultation room/corner). |
| Ich werde mit Ihnen einen Fragebogen durchgehen, um zum Beispiel mögliche Wechselwirkungen auszuschließen. | I will go through this questionnaire with you to make sure that I can exclude possible interactions for example. |
| Ihre Identität bleibt anonym. | Your identity remains anonymous. |
| Weshalb möchten Sie die »Pille danach« kaufen? | Why would you like to purchase the emergency pill? |
| Barrieremethoden | barrier method |
| Empfängnisschutz/Kontrazeption | contraception |
| Nehmen Sie zurzeit ein Kontrazeptivum ein? | Are you currently taking any contraceptive/Are you on birth control? |
| Haben Sie vergessen, eine Pille einzunehmen? | Have you missed a pill? |
| Was ist der Name Ihrer Pille/ihres Kontrazeptivums? | What is the name of your pill/contraceptive? |
| ungeschützter Geschlechtsverkehr | unprotected sex/unprotected sexual intercourse |
| Zeitpunkt | time (of) |
| Wann war der Zeitpunkt des ungeschützten Geschlechtsverkehrs? | When was the time of the unprotected sex? |
| Schwangerschaft | pregnancy |
| Kann eine Schwangerschaft ausgeschlossen werden? | Can you exclude a pregnancy/Are you sure that you are not currently pregnant? |
| Schwangerschaftstest | pregnancy test |
| positiver Schwangerschaftstest | positive pregnancy test |
| XY verzögert oder stoppt den Eisprung. | XY delays or stops the release of an egg/ovulation. |
| Eisprung | ovulation/»release of an egg« |
| nach erfolgtem Eisprung kann eine Schwangerschaft eintreten. | After the ovulation has taken place, a pregnancy can occur. |
| Der Eisprung tritt in der Regel 14 Tage vor Eintreten der Menstruation ein. | The ovulation takes place 14 days before the menstruation begins. |

| | |
|---|---|
| Wann hatten Sie Ihre letzte Monatsblutung? | When was the last time you had your period/menstruation? |
| Ist die letzte Monatsblutung anders ausgefallen als sonst? | Did you notice any changes concerning your last menstruation? |
| Menstruationszyklus | menstrual cycle |
| Zyklusstörungen | menstrual cycle disorders/disturbances |
| Nehmen Sie weitere Medikamente ein? | Do you take any other medication? |
| Neben- und Wechselwirkungen (für typische Nebenwirkungen, die unter der Einnahme von Notfallkontrazeptiva auftreten können ▶ Kap. 3.5.3) | side effects/interactions (s. chapter 3.5.3 for side effects) |
| CYP3A4-Induktoren | CYP3A4-inductors |
| Thrombose(n)/Blutgerinnsel | thrombosis/blood clot |
| Sind innerhalb Ihrer Familie Thrombosen bekannt? | Are any cases of thrombosis known within your family? |
| Kontraindikation | contraindication |
| XY vermeidet und schützt nicht vor sexuellen Krankeiten. | XY does not prevent or protect against sexual diseases. |
| bedenklich | alarming/critical/concerning |
| keine Abgabe auf Vorrat | no dispense in advance |
| Nehmen Sie die Pille so schnell wie möglich ein. | Take the pill as soon as possible. |
| Wirksamkeit | effectiveness |
| Falls Sie innerhalb der nächsten 3 Stunden erbrechen oder starken Durchfall haben, müssen Sie eine weitere Tablette einnehmen. | In case you have to vomit or have diarrhoea within the next 3 hours, you have to take another pill. |
| Stillen | breastfeeding/nursing |
| *Levonorgestrel* | *levonorgestrel* |
| *Ulipristalacetat* | *ulipristal acetate* |
| Intrauterinpessar (»Kupferspirale«) | intrauterine device (ICD/IUCD) |
| XY kann nicht als normale Kontrazeption genommen werden. | XY is not intended to be taken as a regular form of contraception. |
| In Ihrem Falle empfehle ich Ihnen, XY zu nehmen. | In your case I recommend to take XY. |
| In Ihrem Falle brauchen Sie keine Notfallkontrazeption. | In your case you do not need to take an emergency contraceptive. |
| In Ihrem Falle rate ich Ihnen, zum gynäkologischen Bereitschaftsdienst zu gehen. | |

## II Die Beratung – The consultation

|  | In your case, unfortunately, I have to advise you to go to the gynaecological emergency service. |
|---|---|
| gynäkologischer Bereitschaftsdienst | gynaecological emergency service |
| ärztlicher Bereitschaftsdienst | emergency medical service |

**Beispiel – example**

C: *Hello. I need the morning-after pill.*
Y: *Hello. I have to ask you a few questions in order to check whether the emergency pill is suitable for you. Please follow me to our consultation room.*

K: *Hallo. Ich brauche die »Pille danach«.*
S: *Hallo. Ich muss Ihnen einige Fragen stellen, um zu prüfen, ob die Notfall-Pille für Sie geeignet ist. Bitte folgen Sie mir in den Beratungsraum.*

# 6 Sonstiges – Miscellaneous

## 6.1 Baby-Artikel und -Beschwerden – Baby products and ailments

In Kap. 6.1 sind einige Artikel rund um das Thema Baby aufgelistet. Zudem sind auch einige typische Säuglingsbeschwerden dargestellt.

In chapter 6.1 you will find terms for baby articles and ailments.

Baby-Artikel – Baby articles

| | |
|---|---|
| Baby-Körperpflegeartikel/Toilettenartikel | baby toiletries |
| Babybürste | baby brush |
| Babylöffel | baby spoon |
| Babynahrung | baby food |
| Babypuder | baby powder |
| Babyseife | baby soap |
| Bindehautentzündung | conjunctivitis/eye inflammation |
| Dehnungsstreifen | stretch marks |
| Fieberzäpfchen | fever suppository |
| Kolbenspritze | bulb syringe |
| Koliken | colics |
| Milchpumpe | breast pump |
| Nasensauger/Sekretsauger | nasal aspirator |
| Schnabeltasse | sippy cub |
| Schnuller | pacifier |
| Schürfwunden | abrasions/scrapes |
| Schwangerschaft | pregnancy |
| Stillzeit | breastfeeding period/nursing period |

II Die Beratung – The consultation

| Wärmekissen | heat cushion/heat pillow |
| --- | --- |
| Waschhandschuh/Abwaschlappen | washcloth |
| Wickeldecke | swaddle blanket |
| Windelcreme | diaper cream |
| Windeldermatitis | diaper dermatitis/diaper rash |
| Zahnungsbeschwerden | teething problems |
| Zahnungsgel | teething gel |

**Beispiel – example**

C: *I think my child is teething. The gums are a bit red and swollen. She also cries more frequently now.*
K: Ich denke, dass mein Kind zahnt. Das Zahnfleisch ist ein wenig rot und angeschwollen. Sie weint seitdem auch häufiger.

## 6.2 Tierarzneimittel/-artikel – Veterinary medicines/items

Die untenstehenden Artikel/Beschwerden beziehen sich hauptsächlich auf Hunde und Katzen. Deren Besitzer gehören zu den Tierhaltern, die am häufigsten eine Apotheke aufsuchen.

The terms below mainly concern items for and ailments of dogs and cats. Their owners belong to the majority of pet owners, who seek advice in a community pharmacy.

Tierarzneimittel – Veterenary Medicine

| Abwehrmittel | deterrent |
| --- | --- |
| Entwurmungstablette | worming tablets |
| Fliegenabwehrmittel/Fliegenschutzmittel | fly repellent |
| Floh | flea |
| Flohbefallbehandlung (orale) | (oral) flea treatment |
| Flohhalsband | flea collar |
| Flohspray | flea spray |

| | |
|---|---|
| Laus-Repellent/lausabweisendes Mittel | louse repellent |
| Läuse | lice |
| Nagelknipser | nail clipper |
| Ohrreiniger | ear cleaners |
| Wurmmittel | wormers/vermifuge |
| Zecke | tick |
| Zeckenentferner (z. B. Zeckenzange) | tick remover |
| Zeckenhalsband | tick collar |

**Beispiel – example**

C: Since the tick season has started I need a tick collar for my dog.
K: Da die Zeckensaison angefangen hat, brauche ich ein Zeckenhalsband für meinen Hund.

## 6.3 Fachärzte – Medical specialists

Falls Sie einem Patienten mit Verdacht auf Hämorrhoiden sagen wollen, dass er sich am besten von einem Proktologen untersuchen lassen sollte, dann werden Sie hier fündig. Diese Liste stellt lediglich eine Auswahl an Facharztrichtungen dar.

In case you need to explain to a patient suspected of having haemorrhoids that he or she should see a proctologist, you will find relevant expressions here. This table represents only a selection of medical specialists.

(Fach-)Ärzte – Medical specialists (selection)

| | |
|---|---|
| Facharzt | specialist physician (AF)/medical specialist |
| Allergologe | allergist/immunologist |
| Augenarzt | ophthalmologist |
| Gynäkologe | gynaecologist |
| Hals-Nasen-Ohren-Arzt | otolaryngologist |

| | |
|---|---|
| (Haus-)Arzt/Facharzt für Allgemeinmedizin | physician (AE)/general practicioner (GP) (BE), medical doctor (NZ)/specialist for general medicine |
| Hautarzt | dermatologist |
| Internist/Facharzt für Inneres | internist |
| Kardiologe | cardiologist |
| Kinderarzt | pediatrician/paediatrician |
| Nephrologe | nephrologist |
| Neurologe | neurologist |
| Nuklearmediziner | nuclear medicine practitioner |
| Orthopäde | orthopedist (AE)/othopaedist (BE) |
| Proktologe | proctologist |
| Psychiater | psychiatrist |
| Chirurg | surgeon |
| Tropenmediziner | physician for tropical medicine |
| Urologe | urologist |
| Zahnarzt | dentist |

**Beispiel – example**

Y: *If you suspect to suffer from haemorrhoids (BE) you should go and see a proctologist.*
S: Falls Sie den Verdacht haben, an Hämorrhoiden zu leiden, sollten Sie zu einem Proktologen gehen.

## 6.4 Andere Gesundheitsberufe – Other health care professions

| | |
|---|---|
| Arzthelfer | physician assistant/physician associate |
| Chiropraktiker | chiropractor |
| Ergotherapeut | occupational therapist |
| Ernährungsberater | dietician |
| Hebamme | midwife |

| | |
|---|---|
| Krankenschwester/-pfleger | nurse |
| Logopäde | speech therapist |
| Optiker | optician/optometrist |
| Physiotherapeut | physical therapist |
| Podologe | podiatrist |
| Psychologe | psychologist |
| Rettungssanitäter | emergency medical technician |

**Beispiel – example**

C: *Both my GP and midwife recommended to substitute folic acid during pregnancy. Do you have any small packages?*
S: *Mein Arzt und meine Hebamme haben mir empfohlen, Folsäure während der Schwangerschaft zu substituieren. Haben Sie kleine Packungen da?*

## 6.5 Die Wochentage – Weekdays

| | |
|---|---|
| Montag | Monday |
| Dienstag | Tuesday |
| Mittwoch | Wednesday |
| Donnerstag | Thursday |
| Freitag | Friday |
| Samstag | Saturday |
| Sonntag | Sunday |

**Beispiel – example**

Y: *Our opening times are Monday to Friday from 8 a.m. until 6 p.m.*
S: *Unsere Öffnungszeiten sind Montag bis Freitag von 8 bis 18 Uhr.*

II Die Beratung – The consultation

## 6.6 Uhrzeiten – Times of the day

| | |
|---|---|
| Nachmittag (12:00 Uhr bis 23:59 Uhr) | p.m. = post meridiem |
| Vormittag (0:00 Uhr bis 11:59 Uhr) | a.m. = ante meridiem |
| halb XY (im Englischen eine halbe Stunde nach XY) *Beispiel: halb 12 (= 11:30)* | half past XY *example: half past 11 (= 11:30)* |
| Viertel nach XY | a quarter past |
| Viertel vor XY | a quarter to XY |

Da Sie im Englischen a.m. oder p.m. als Zeitangabe hinzufügen, verwenden Sie immer die gleichen Zahlen. Es erfolgt somit keine Unterscheidung der Uhrzeitzahlen wie im Deutschen.

| | |
|---|---|
| 13 Uhr | 1 p.m. |
| 1 Uhr | 1 a.m. |

**Beispiel – example**

Y: *It is a quarter past 9 a.m.*
S: Es ist viertel nach 9 Uhr.

# III Nicht pharmazeutische Anliegen – Non-pharmacy related matters

# 7 Anliegen und Begriffe – Matters and terms

Fast jeden Tag kommen Kunden mit nicht-pharmazeutischen Anliegen in die Apotheke. Sie wollen zum Beispiel den Weg zum nächsten Bahnhof wissen oder, ob Sie Haargummis verkaufen. Da dies oft genug vorkommt, ist dieser Teil ebenfalls enthalten.

Almost every day patients inquire about non-pharmacy related matters in the community pharmacy. They ask for directions to the next train station for instance or whether you sell hair ties. Since you will encounter these non-pharmaceutical matters frequently this chapter has also been included in this book.

## 7.1 Wegbeschreibungen – Directions

| | |
|---|---|
| Ampel | traffic light |
| Arztpraxis | doctor's office/medical surgery/medical office/doctor's practice |
| Bahnhof | train station |
| Bank | bank |
| Bibliothek | library |
| bis | until |
| Botschaft | embassy |
| Bushaltestelle | bus stop |
| der/die/das nächste | the next/nearest |
| der Straße folgen | to follow the road |
| Flughafen | airport |
| Geldautomat | ATM (automated teller machine) |
| geradeaus gehen | to go straight ahead |
| Ich müsste/muss zum/zur XY gehen. | I need to go to the XY. |

### III Nicht pharmazeutische Anliegen – Non-pharmacy related matters

| | |
|---|---|
| in eine Straße fahren | to enter a road |
| Können Sie mir sagen, wo der/ die/das nächste XY ist? | Can you tell me where the next XY is? |
| Könnten Sie mir sagen, wo die nächste/n XY ist? | Could you please explain to me where the next XY is? |
| Krankenhaus | hospital |
| Kreisel/Kreisverkehr | roundabout |
| öffentliche Toilette | public restroom (AE)/public toilet |
| Polizeistation | police station |
| Post | post office |
| Rathaus | town council/town hall |
| rechts/links abbiegen | to turn right/left |
| Sanitätshaus | health care supply store/medical supply store |
| Schild | sign |
| Schule | school |
| Straßenbahn | tram |
| steuerfrei | tax free |
| Supermarkt | supermarket |
| U-Bahn | subway (AE)/underground (BE) |
| Universität | university |
| Wo ist XY? | Where is a/the XY? |

### Beispiel – example

*C: Excuse me, can you tell me where the next bus station is?*
*Y: Follow the road until you see the first stop sign. Then turn right.*

K: Entschuldigung, können Sie mir sagen, wo die nächste Bushaltestelle ist?
S: Folgen Sie der Straße bis Sie das erste Stopschild sehen. Danach müssen Sie rechts abbiegen.

## 7.2 Nicht pharmazeutische Gegenstände – Non-pharmacy related items

| | |
|---|---|
| Badelatschen/Flip-Flops | flip-flops/bathing shoes/jandals* |
| Haarklammer | bobby pin |
| Kamm/Haarbürste | comb/hair brush |
| Lippenstift | lipstick |
| Nagelfeile | nail file |
| Parfüm | perfume |
| Rasiercreme | shaving cream |
| Rasiergel | shaving gel |
| Rasierklinge | razor |
| Rasierpinsel | shaving brush |
| Rasierschaum | shaving foam |
| Sicherheitsnadeln | safety pins |
| Sonnenbrille | sun glasses |

\* In Neuseeland heißen Flip-Flops jandals.

### Beispiel – example

Y: *I am sorry, but we do not sell sunglasses.*
S: Es tut mir leid, aber wir verkaufen keine Sonnenbrillen.

## 7.3 Keine Auskunft möglich – Provision of information not possible

| | |
|---|---|
| Es tut mir leid, aber ich weiß nicht, wo XY ist. | I am afraid, I do not know where XY is. |
| Es tut mir leid, aber ich kenne mich in der Umgebung auch nicht aus. | I am sorry, I am not familiar with the surroundings. |
| Es tut mir leid, aber ich kann Ihnen nicht helfen. | I am sorry, but I cannot help you. |
| Ich könnte allerdings meine Kollegen fragen, ob die wissen, wo XY ist. | I could ask my colleagues, however, if they know where XY is. |

III Nicht pharmazeutische Anliegen – Non-pharmacy related matters

| Wenn Sie wünschen, kann ich meine Kollegen fragen, ob die wissen, wo XY ist. | If you wish, I could ask my colleagues if they know where XY is. |

### Beispiel – example

*Y: I am afraid, I do not know if there is a copy shop nearby.*
S: Es tut mir leid, aber ich weiß nicht, ob es einen Copyshop in der Nähe gibt.

**IV** Online-Zusatzmaterial und Wörterverzeichnis – Electronic supplementary material and vocabulary index

# 8 Zusatzmaterial zum Download – Electronic supplementary material

Die Zusatzmaterialien[10] können Sie unter folgendem Link herunterladen:
You can access the supplementary material by clicking on the following link:

https://dl.kohlhammer.de/978-3-17-041138-8

---

10 Wichtiger urheberrechtlicher Hinweis: Alle zusätzlichen Materialien, die im Download-Bereich zur Verfügung gestellt werden, sind urheberrechtlich geschützt. Ihre Verwendung ist nur zum persönlichen und nichtgewerblichen Gebrauch erlaubt. Jede Verwendung außerhalb der engen Grenzen des Urheberrechts ist ohne Zustimmung des Verlags unzulässig und strafbar. Das gilt insbesondere für Vervielfältigungen, Übersetzungen, Mikroverfilmungen und für die Einspeicherung und Verarbeitung in elektronischen Systemen.

# Wörterverzeichnis – Index

## A

Anwendung – administration
- Anwendungsart – route of administration  54, 55
- Anwendungshinweise – administration directions  55–58, 71, 90
- Einnahmezeitpunkt – time of intake  56
- Nach der Mahlzeit – after a meal/postprandial  56
- Nüchtern – on an empty stomach/sober  56
- Peroral/oral – peroral/oral  54
- Topisch – topical  55

Apotheke – pharmacy
- Krankenhaus-Apotheke – hospital pharmacy  82
- Öffentliche Apotheke – community pharmacy/retail pharmacy  81, 82

Arzneimittel – medicine
- Tierarzneimittel – veterinary medicines  47, 118, 119
- Verschreibungsfreie – nonprescription  47, 83, 95, 100, 101, 105, 115
- Verschreibungspflichtige – prescription only  32–47, 86, 88–91

Aufbrauchfrist – grace period  65

## B

Beipackzettel – package leaflet  48
Belieferung – delivery/supply  81
Beratung (allgemein) – consultation (in general)  57, 58, 77–79, 81, 82, 90, 91
Bioverfügbarkeit – bioavailability  63
Blutspiegeländerung – change in blood level  26, 60, 63

## D

Darreichungsform – dosage form
- Feste Darreichungsformen – solid dosage forms  50
- Kapsel – capsule  50
- Tablette – tablet  50
- Flüssige Darreichungsformen – liquid dosage forms  51
- Augentropfen – eye drops  51
- Lösung – solution  51
- Halbfeste Darreichungsformen – semi solid dosage forms  51
- Creme – cream  51
- Gel – gel  51
- Salbe – salve  51
- Zäpfchen – suppository  51
- Inhalatoren – inhalers  52

Dosierung – dosage/dose  57
- Dosieranweisung – dosing instructions  57
- Dosisanpassung – dose adjustment  57

## E

Einnahmedauer – intake duration  56, 87

## F

Facharzt – specialist physician (AE)/medical specialist  119, 120
Fachinformation – drug label/summary of product characteristics  48

## G

Genehmigung beantragen – apply for approval  88
Generikum – generic drug  89
Großhändler – wholesale supplier  89

## H

Haltbarkeit – shelf life  65

133

## K

Komissionierer/einrichtungsbezogene Begriffe – pharmacy robot/furniture-related terms   82
Kontraindikation – contraindication   48, 115
Krankenversicherung – health insurance   87–90
Krankheiten – diseases   19–24, 111, 112

## L

Lagerung – storage
- Lagerungshinweise – storage information   48, 58, 64–66
- Temperaturen – temperatures   64

Löslichkeit – solubility   32, 53

## N

Nebenwirkung – side effect   31, 49, 58–61, 115
- Häufigkeit – frequency   59, 60
- Schweregrad – severity   59

## P

Patient(-engruppe) – patient(-group)   49
Pflanzen/Phytotherapeutika – plants/phytotherapeutics   66–69
Produktklasse – product type   47
- Hilfsmittel – therapeutic appliance   47
- Medizinprodukt – medicinal product   47
- Nahrungsergänzungsmittel – nutritional supplement   47

## R

Reiseimpfungen und -krankheiten – travel vaccinations and diseases   21, 22, 108–112
Rezept – prescription   87–90
- Betäubungsmittelrezept – controlled substance prescription   88
- Empfehlungsrezept – recommendation/OTC-prescription   88
- Entlassrezept – discharge prescription   88
- Erstattung – reimbursement   89
- Kassenrezept – panel prescription   88
- Privatrezept – private prescription   88
- Rezeptgebühr – prescription charge   89
- Zuzahlungsbefreiung – copayment exempt   88

Rezepturen – pharmaceutical compounding   71, 72
- Herstellungsdatum – date of manufacture   71
- Inkompatibilität – incompatibility   71

## S

Selbstmedikation – self-medication   83–85
- Erkältung – common cold   92, 93
- Grenzen der Selbstmedikation – self-medication limits   85, 86
- Husten – cough   93–99
- Notfallkontrazeption – emergency contraception   113–115
- Schmerzen – ache/pain   28, 94, 98, 105–109
- Schnupfen – blocked nose   98–102

Symptom/Beschwerde – symptom/complaint   25–29, 57, 79–81, 92, 93, 96–100, 103, 104, 109
- Blähungen – flatulence   26
- Durchfall – diarrhea (AE)/diarrhoea (BE)   26, 60, 62, 115
- Erbrechen – vomit   26, 104, 115
- Fieber – fever   21, 22, 26, 92, 94, 109, 112
- Haarausfall – hair-loss   25, 26
- Halsweh – sore throat   26, 29
- Heiserkeit – hoarseness   26, 94
- Insektenstich – insect bite   27
- Juckreiz – itch   27, 80
- Menstruationsbeschwerden – menstrual complaints   27, 103
- Müdigkeit – tiredness   27, 61
- Schmerz – pain   28, 94, 98, 106, 108, 109
- Sodbrennen – heartburn   28, 96
- Übelkeit – nausea   28, 62, 104
- Veränderungen des Blutdrucks – change in blood pressure   21, 26, 60, 61, 85, 86
- Verstopfung – constipation   28
- Warze – verruca/wart   29

## T

Tablettenbox – tablet storage box   65
Tablettenteiler – tablet cutter/splitter   58

## V

Verbandstoff – wound dressing   73
Verfalldatum – expiry date   65, 66

## W

Wechselwirkung – interaction 49, 58, 62, 63, 114, 115
Wirksamkeit – efficacy (unter Idealbedingungen), effectiveness (unter Routinebedingungen) 31, 49, 63, 115
Wirkstoff – active ingredient 72, 91, 97, 100, 105, 107
- Wirkort – site of action/target location 31
- Wirkstofffreisetzung – drug release 31, 53, 54, 62
Wirkstoffklasse – drug class 32–46, 95
- Analgetikum/Schmerzmittel – analgesic/pain killer 32, 36, 104
- Antazida – antacids 33
- Antiallergika – antiallergics 33
- Antibiotikum – antibiotic 35, 36, 46, 64
- Antidiabetika – antidiabetics 34, 35
- Antidiarrhoika – antidiarrheals (AE)/antidiarrhoeals (BE) 35
- Antihistaminikum – antihistamine 33, 35, 44
- Antiinfektiva – antiinfectives 36
- Antikonvulsiva – anticonvulsive agents 38
- Antimigräne-Mittel – antimigraine agents 36
- Antimykotika – antimycotics 37
- Antithrombose-Mittel – antithrombotic agents
- Digestiva – digestives 40
- Herz-Kreislauf-Mittel – cardiovascular agents 41
- Hormone – hormones 42, 45, 46
- Immunsuppressiva – immunosuppressants 40
- Insulin – insulin 24, 58
- Laxanzien – laxatives 42
- Osteoporose-Mittel – osteoporosis treatment agents 44
- Psychopharmaka – psychopharmacologic drugs 44
- Virustatika – antivirals
- Vitamine – vitamins 38, 44, 45
- Zytostatika – cytostatics 40, 46